INTRAOPERATIVE ULTRASONOGRAPHY IN HEPATO-BILIARY AND
PANCREATIC SURGERY

SERIES IN RADIOLOGY

Volume 19

Intraoperative Ultrasonography in Hepato-Biliary and Pancreatic Surgery

A Practical Guide

Edited by

GIUSEPPE GOZZETTI & ALIGHIERI MAZZIOTTI

Department of Surgery, University of Bologna

LUIGI BOLONDI & LUIGI BARBARA

Department of Medicine, University of Bologna

With contributions by

YVES CHAPUIS

Department of Surgery, Hôpital Cochin, Paris

JEAN-FRANÇOIS GIGOT & PAUL-JACQUES KESTENS

Department of Surgery, University of Louvain, Bruxelles

Kluwer Academic Publishers

Dordrecht / Boston / London

Library of Congress Cataloging in Publication Data

Intraoperative ultrasonography in hepato-biliary and pancreatic surgery
  : a practical guide / edited by Giuseppe Gozzetti ... [et al.] ;
with contributions by Yves Chapuis, Jean Francois Gigot, Paul
Jacques Kestens.
        p.   cm. -- (Series in radiology)
    Translated from Italian.
    Includes bibliographies and index.

    1. Liver--Surgery. 2. Biliary tract--Surgery. 3. Pancreas-
-Surgery. 4. Operative ultrasonography.   I. Gozzetti, Giuseppe.
II. Chapuis, Y. III. Gigot, Jean Francois.   IV. Kestens, P.-J.
(Paul-J.) V. Series,.
    [DNLM: 1. Biliary'Tract Surgery. 2. Intraoperative Care.
3. Liver--surgery. 4. Pancreas--surgery. 5. Ultrasonic Diagnosis-
-methods.   WI 770 I61]
RD546.I59 1989
617.5'56059--dc20
DNLM/DLC
for Library of Congress   89-15267

ISBN-13: 978-94-010-6924-3   e-ISBN-13: 978-94-009-0967-0
DOI: 10.1007/978-94-009-0967-0

Published by Kluwer Academic Publishers,
P.O. Box 17, 3300 AA Dordrecht, The Netherlands

Kluwer Academic Publishers incorporates
the publishing programmes of
D. Reidel, Martinus Nijhoff, Dr w. Junk and MTP Press.

Sold and distributed in the U.S.A. and Canada
by Kluwer Academic Publishers,
101 Philip Drive, Norwell, MA 02061, U.S.A.

In all other countries, sold and distributed
by Kluwer Academic Publishers Group,
P.O. Box 322, 3300 AH Dordrecht, The Netherlands.

Translated by Mrs Stephanie Johnson

Original edition: Ecografia intraoperatoria in chirurgia epato-biliare e pancreatica.
© Masson, S.p.A., Milan, 1986.

Printed on acid free paper

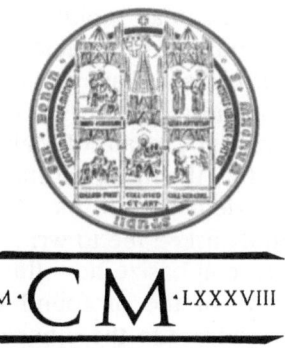

M·C M·LXXXVIII

Alma Mater Studiorum
Sæcularia Nona

Foreword

In 1983 and 1984, I had the pleasure of being invited to Europe for the Course of Hepatobiliary Surgery started by Professor Hepp and continued by Professor Bismuth. In these courses, I demonstrated many slides and movies of intraoperative echography that Makuuchi, one of my staff members, had made using the transducer that he was the first to develop.

The topic of Intraoperative Echography had an enormous impact on the audience, and its use has since spread rapidly over the European countries, by virtue of the first Italian edition of Professor Gozzetti's book on Intraoperative Echography and Professor Bismuth's monograph on the same topic. I had been, therefore, unwittingly a very fortunate transmitter of intraoperative echography to Europe by means of Makuuchi's slide file.

I am extremely honoured that the Italian Edition written by Gozzetti, Mazziotti and Bolondi has been dedicated to me. Also in this English Edition, Professor Gozzetti very kindly asked me to write a few words. It is an extraordinary pleasure for me to emphasize how this book is easy to read and understand, maybe by virtue of the profound Italian tradition of artistic expression since the Renaissance. On the other hand, a variety of series of intraoperative echographic images as well as resected specimens are arranged in an excellent manner. The work covers not only primary and metastatic lesions but also bile duct lesions as well as portal hypertension and liver transplantation. The schematic presentation of transducer use know-how during surgery is also unique.

All in all, this book will help not only young surgeons from the view point of easy accessibility and clarity, but will also help well-trained surgeons because of the valuable information included in the images and descriptive text.

Hiroshi Hasegawa
Professor of Surgery
National Cancer Center Hospital
Tokyo
December 1988

Foreword

The advent of intraoperative ultrasonography (IOU) not only changed the attitude of the surgeon towards many important intra-abdominal diseases but also produced substantial improvements in surgical technique. In major hepatobiliary centers wordwide, some operations on the liver pancreas and bile ducts are no longer performed without the help and guide of this new method. This is particularly true in surgery of liver neoplasms where IOU permits recognition of very small nodules and limited resections especially in cirrhotic livers.

Small hepatic metastates are often missed by conventional imaging modalities due either to insufficient resolution of the technique or due to the particular location of the lesion. Careful IOU survey during surgical exploration for primary gastrointestinal malignancies may discover unsuspected metastatic nodules which can then be easily resected under guidance of the ultrasound probe.

Hepatocellular carcinoma complicating cirrhosis constitutes perhaps the best indication for IOU. The search for a small neoplastic nodule within the firm and hard cirrhotic liver parenchyma is frustrating and often benefits from the application of an intraoperative ultrasound probe to locate non palpable nodules. In addition, preservation of functioning liver tissue is an important surgical goal in such patients in order to protect liver metabolic reserve. IOU makes it possible to produce a clearcut display of hepatic vascular anatomy and of the relationship between tumor and potential resection planes.

In biliary surgery the search for calculi or the exact definition of neoplastic infiltration are greatly facilitated by IOU and in some instances this technique is preferred to the more traditional intraoperative cholangiography.

Lastly, surgery for endocrine tumors of the pancreas can simply not be accurately carried out without the use of intra-operative ultrasound guidance to detect small non-palpable nodules Embedded in the glandular tissue.

All of these topics, and many others, have been extensively reviewed in this volume based on the impressive clinical experience of these European authors. Each clinical problem is presented within its medical and surgical context and illustrated by high quality sonographic images.

The book may serve either as a basic introduction to the role of intraoperative ultrasound for surgeons or as a useful complimentary source of information for those who are already well versed in abdominal ultrasonography and wish to pursue intra-operative applications. Thus, physicians with a background in surgery, gastroenterology and radiology are all likely to benefit from the new knowledge presented in this fine volume.

Joseph T. Ferrucci, M.D.
Professor of Radiology
Harvard Medical School
Boston
March 1989

Preface

Recent years have seen an increasing use of intraoperative ultrasound which has now become a routine procedure in an ever growing number of centers.

The use of high frequency, high resolution probes, along with the possibility of directly investigating the vessels and ducts of the organ in question make intraoperative ultrasound an important aid to ensure radical, safer surgery. The aim of the investigation is to detect the presence or absence of lesions and their location with regard to adjacent vessels, as well as provide an overall assessment of the lesion's extension. All this information can be obtained immediately, at the outset of surgery, thereby avoiding exploratory tissue dissection, traumatic surgical manoeuvers and the use of contrast medium.

First employed in urology and vascular surgery and subsequently, with the development of real time equipment, in biliary surgery, intraoperative ultrasound is today most widely used in surgery involving the abdominal parenchimal organs, i.e. the liver and pancreas. Inspection and palpation – methods that often fail to pick up deep lesions and are especially precarious in the presence of liver cirrhosis, chronic pancreatitis or organs having undergone previous surgery – may be flanked and perfected by the use of intraoperative ultrasonography. Intra-parenchymal lesions of even less than one centimetre are easily detected while the vascular configuration of each patient can be mapped, thereby ensuring safer, easier dissection. Also detectable are areas where the lesion compresses or infiltrates the intra or extra-parenchymal vessels along with the presence of neoplastic thrombi even in small branches. In fact intraoperative ultrasonography is of particular use in surgery for hepatic tumours and was initially used in Far Eastern countries where hepatocarcinoma is very prevalent. Indeed most of the credit goes to Professors Hiroshi Hasegawa and Masatoshi Makuuchi for developing brillant ultrasound techniques during hepatic resection. During their lecture tour in 1983–84, these two surgeons presented revolutionary images during liver surgery, showing us that we can actually look inside the liver,identifying the relations between pathological mass and the hepato-portal vascular peduncles. Prof. Henri Bismuth of Villejuif in France was the first to understand the importance of this new approach, followed by ourselves in Italy along with other groups in Europe.

In our experience intraoperative ultrasound has been mainly used during surgery for liver tumors. We therefore wanted to present our data in greater detail with this book.

Intraoperative ultrasound is also being applied to great advantage in bilary surgery, both for lithiasis and tumors. In the case of the former there are conflicting views among surgeons, some preferring ultrasound to intraoperative cholangiography while others maintain that intraoperative ultrasonography merely complements conventional investigations and should be used only in particular circumstances. In order to provide an objective view we have sought the collaboration of a highly experienced group of biliary surgeons, namely Professor Kestens and Dr Gigot of Brussels.

Intraoperative ultrasound is proving of use also in pancreatic surgery, in particular the search for endocrine tumors. We are honoured to have the contribution of Professor Chapuis of Paris for this chapter.

With the development of the Doppler transducers new possibilities are being opened up to measure blood flow in the visceral vessels. The major application here is in portal shunt surgery and more recently, organ transplantation.

During intraoperation surgery the major difficulty facing the surgeon is getting used to the ultrasonic image, recognizing the appearance of lesions and taking care to conduct the scanning planes accurately. The bidimensional data of ultrasonography must be considered in their spatial context, along with 'gain', contrast and grey scale. Here we have received enormous support from the long standing collaboration between our surgical team and the Ultrasound Group of the Department of Medicine at the University of Bologna. Working together with Luigi Bolondi of Professor Barbara's department has been both fruitful and stimulating. Indeed it is largely thanks to their encouragement and enthusiasm that intraoperative ultasonography has become a routine investigation during hepatobiliary and pancreatic surgery. This book is intended as a practical guide to anyone preparing to use ultrasonography intraoperatively. The wide range of ultrasonic images has been chosen with the surgeon in mind and accompanied by radiological data and pictures of operative specimens.

This book is an updated reprint of a first edition published in 1986 by Masson Italia. This English edition has been requested by Kluwer Academic Publishers to allow for wider distribution.

Giuseppe Gozzetti
December 1988
Bologna

Abbreviations and diagrams

The following abbreviations have been used in the echographic photographs and in the diagrams. In these latter the position and orientation of the probe is often indicated.

a: aorta
bd: biliary duct
an: angioma
cbd: common bile duct
cl: caudate lobe
d: duodenum
df: diaphragm
gb: gallbladder
gda: gastro duodenal artery
ha: hepatic artery
hd: hepatic (bile) duct
hem: hematoma
hv: hepatic vein
k: kidney
l: liver
lhd: left hepatic duct
lo: lesser omentum
lpv: left branch of the portal vein
lra: left renal artery

m: metastasis
mhv: middle hepatic vein
n: needle
p: pancreas
pv: portal vein
pbr: portal branch
rhd: right hepatic (biliary) duct
rhv: right hepatic vein
rpv: right branch of the portal vein
rv: renal vein
s: stone
sa: splenic artery
sma: superior mesenteric artery
st: stomach
sv: splenic vein
t: tumor
vc: vena cava
w: Wirsung duct

Table of contents

CHAPTER 9: INTRAOPERATIVE ULTRASOUND DURING SURGERY FOR PORTAL HYPERTENSION AND LIVER TRANSPLANTATION

Chapter 1: Physical principles and instrumentation

The physics of ultrasound

Sound waves can be defined as mechanical oscillations made to pass through a solid, liquid or gaseous medium. As wave propagation is caused by the movement of particles, it follows that no transmission occurs through a vacuum. The passage of sound waves entails pressure variations in the medium i.e. alternating positive and negative pressures. *Wavelength* (λ) indicates one complete cycle accomplished by a wave passing through positive and negative positions. Wavelength multiplied by *frequency* i.e. the number of full cycles per second, gives the *velocity (C) of sound*: $F \times \lambda = C$. As velocity is constant in a given medium at a given temperature, frequency and wavelength are inversely proportional.

Frequency is measured in Hertz (Hz) and indicates the number of cycles per second (cps).

Ultrasound waves are sound waves with a frequency exceeding 20 KHz, which is the highest frequency audible to the human ear. For diagnostic purposes the frequency range commonly used is between 1 to 10 MHz (1 MHz = 10 Hz) [2].

The *intensity* of the ultrasound waves passing through living tissue is all-important. Intensity is measured in Watt/cm^2 and expresses the pressure exerted by the ultrasound wave per unit area. In other words, intensity indicates the amount of energy transmitted by the ultrasound beam.

Another order of magnitude related to intensity, and frequently referred to in ultrasonics, is the *decibel (dB)*. 1 dB = 10 log 10 (l/Io) where I is the intensity of the particular ultrasound beam and Io a reference intensity. Decibels are often used to express the magnitude of the echoes generated when ultrasound waves pass through tissues. Since intensity is directly proportional to the square of wave *amplitude*, it follows that 1 dB = 20 log 10 (A/Ao), where A is the amplitude of the reflected wave or echo and Ao is the amplitude of the incident wave.

Ultrasound wave generation

Ultrasound equipment makes use of the *piezoelectric effect*. This is the capacity of certain crystals (eg. quartz) or certain ceramic materials (eg. lead zirconate and barium titanate) to vibrate at exactly the same frequency when subjected to an alternating current. When electric oscillations syncronize with the oscillation characteristic of the crystal excited, the phenomenon of resonance occurs and the crystal vibrates at peak amplitude. The result is suitably powerful beams of ultrasound waves produced even by low voltages. The piezoelectric effect is also reversible. If the very same wave-emitting crystal is subjected to the mechanical pressure exerted by an echo, it will generate a voltage that is directly proportional to the pressure applied. If electrodes are then applied to the crystal, the voltage can be recorded and measured. In fact ultrasound probes have the dual function of both emitting the ultrasound beam and picking up the returning echoes. The frequency of the wave generated by the piezoelectric effect depends largely on the ceramic used: when ceramic is subject to an electrical impulse the resultant ultrasound beam has a wide frequency spectrum. In fact although nominal frequency usually refers to the peak frequency, an ultrasound beam comprises several frequencies. Probes are made up of a number of crystals and will have a predetermined nominal frequency. If different working frequencies are required, different probes must be employed.

Interaction between ultrasound waves and tissue

The specific properties of biological tissue affect the transmission of ultrasound waves. Ultrasonic *velocity* varies considerably depending on whether the medium is air, bone or soft tissue. In liver, kidney and blood, velocity is approximately 1540 m/sec with slight variations for specific soft tissue. Tissue *density* can be said to relate both to the atomic number of its components and to physical state. Living tissue has a further property essential for ultrasound: *acoustic impedance*. This is what causes the reflected echo and is the product of the velocity of sound in a given medium multiplied by medium density. Acoustic impedance is fundamental to ultrasound imaging and is a function not only of density (an all-important feature for radiologic imaging) but also of sound velocity through tissue. Therefore, it can be readily understood how lesions that are isodense or of equal density at CT Scan, show up clearly at ultrasound.

Every time an ultrasound wave impinges upon the boundary or interface dividing two media of different acoustic impedance, it loses part of its energy in the form of a reflected wave. This is the echo that is picked up by the ultrasound probe. The amount of energy reflected (and recorded as echo amplitude) is minimal when the sound wave passes through media of very similar acoustic impedance. The greater this difference, the greater the energy loss. In sum, there will be as many echoes as there are boundaries dividing heterogeneous tissue or media.

The greater the difference in acoustic impedance of the two media crossed, the greater will be the amplitude of the reflected echo: heterogeneous or echogenic media will generate many echoes while homogeneous, echofree or transonic media will be silent.

The laws of geometrical optics, namely *reflection, refraction* and *diffraction*, are pertinent to ultrasound. Any simple guide to optical physics will provide adequate explanation of these principles. It should be remembered, however, that the intensity of an ultrasonic beam passing through a medium diminishes exponentially as it travels away from the sound-emitting source.

The sound absorption coefficient increases with frequency. Hence the higher the frequency of an ultrasound beam, the greater the sound absorption.

The 'echogenicity' of soft tissues such as kidney, liver or muscle, cannot be fully explained, however, by differences in acoustic impedance, since these are minimal (5%). The reason lies in their *'bulk modulus'*, i.e. elasticity or rigidity (lack of elasticity) which is all-important to a tissue's capacity to generate echoes. Tissue elasticity depends on the amount of collagen, other fibrous proteins and fatty infiltrate; hence it is these substances that play a primary role in determining the echogenicity of tissue [5].

Basically there are two types of echo generated by the passage of ultrasound waves (Fig. 1.1): *specular echoes*, which are very strong and depend on the angle of incidence at which the ultrasound beam hits the echo-emitting interface (eg. diaphragm, spinal column, the capsule enclosing parenchymatous organs) and 2) *scattered echoes*, which vary little with angle of incidence and are generated within parenchyma and soft tissues, giving the so-called 'echopattern or structure'. In these tissues the reflecting surfaces are oriented in all directions. Furthermore the presence of collagen and fatty tissue will determine differing echo amplitudes [6].

Attenuation of the ultrasound beam is the sum of the energy losses due to absorption and the production of specular and scattered echoes. Attenuation

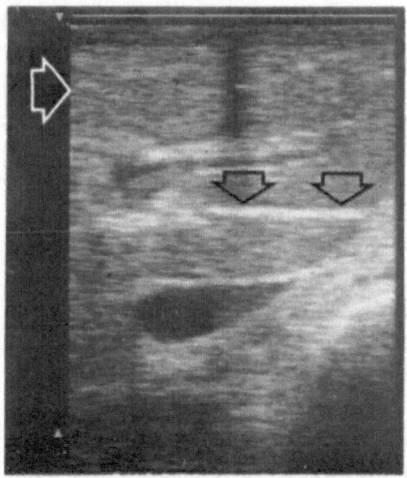

Figure 1.1. This scan of the left lobe of the liver evidences *specular echoes* (black arrows) generated at the interface between the lesser omentum and the caudate lobe. The *scattered echoes* (white arrows) give the typical echo pattern of hepatic parenchyma.

progresses as the beam moves deeper into tissue and is compensated for by an electronic device called a Time Gain Control or TGC. Compensation is exponential to the same extent as attenuation.

Instrumentation

Main features

Ultrasound equipment used in diagnostics comprises the following essential components: a) a *transducer* – a piezoelectric ceramic element mounted on a support. The transducer acts as both transmitter of ultrasound waves at a given frequency and receiver, converting the reflected echoes into electrical signals. All transducers, be they single or multiple crystal, are mounted on a probe. The probe contains the transducer activating systems, namely: b) an *amplifier* to step-up the voltage of the electric signals and c) a signal processing and *imaging* system. Today the B (Brightness)-mode system is used whereby the echoes are represented as points of light. Returning echoes vary widely in amplitude and this amplitude range is imaged by differing tones of grey: high intensity echoes appear white, low intensity echoes gray, while echo-free areas are black. This is the so-called *'grey scale'*. The grey scale range varies from one machine to another and largely determines the quality of the image on the screen. In any one scan the echoes generated will be of variable amplitude within a range of approximately 90 dB. *'Dynamic range'* means the capacity of the ultrasound machine to reproduce the different amplitudes of the echoes generated by tissue. To do this, special systems are employed to compress signals at both ends of the scale (echoes from bone and air) and expand intermediary signals (coming from parenchyma) so that fine structural differences will show up. By *resolution* is meant the machine's capacity to separately image two adjacent interfaces.

Axial resolution is the capacity to distinguish two points on a line parallel to the ultrasound beam as separate sound sources. The higher the frequency and the shorter the ultrasound pulse, the greater the axial resolution. State of the art ultrasound equipment has an axial resolution of approx. 1 mm.

Lateral resolution is the capacity to distinguish at a given distance two points on a line perpendicular to the ultrasound beam. Lateral resolution is a function of beam width, which varies from one type of transducer to another, and especially of beam focussing or focal spot [4]. Lateral resolution will be best (approx. 3 mm) in the focal region but only about 10 mm at more distant points.

Ultrasound beam *focussing* is thus all-important. The beam is focussed either by superimposing acoustic lenses on the transducer or – with linear probes – using electronic systems to sequentially excite the crystals. Both these manoeuvers give *dynamic focussing* virtually along the whole length of the beam axis [3].

Another essential feature of ultrasound equipment is the system of adjustment, known as *gain* setting.

As already noted, the ultrasound beam gradually becomes attenuated the further it travels from the sound-emitting source with the result that, at the same acoustic impedance, returning echoes are of lower amplitude the deeper they originate. To offset this, all ultrasound equipment has an automatic compensation device known as a *Time Gain Control (TGC)*. In short, the TGC amplifies sound even when at considerable depth. Similarly, the returning echoes can be amplified. This amplification is known as 'gain' and modern ultrasound equipment uses a variety of means to achieve 'near' gain to enhance the echoes returning from the more superficial layers or 'far' gain for those coming from tissue at greater depth. Some machines allow differentiated adjustment, centimeter by centimeter, thanks to special cursors. Gain control is indispensable to counter the differing attenuation factors of the various organs or of the individual himself (meterorism, obesity, scars etc.) and ensure high quality, homogeneous images.

Real-time equipment

'Real-time' ultrasonography is particularly indicated for operative applications. The term comes from computer jargon and indicates the sequential representation of dynamic images at a frequency of 16 to 60 images or frames per second [7]. In this way living organs and tissue can be seen as they move with no loss of image on the display screen as the probe is moved about to explore different areas.

Various types of 'real time' equipment are available, the differences lying in the particular probe or transducer used. Probes can be:

1. Linear array probes. Comprising an aligned sequence of 64-400 transducers that are excited in groups. Available probes vary in length from 3 to 12 cm, with an emission frequency ranging from 3.5 to 7.5 MHz.

The resultant images are rectangular and focussing over the whole field of view is dynamic.

Formerly, beam divergence caused by the small size of each single transducer was a problem. Today this has been overcome and the only drawback of this type of probe is its long, inflexible contact surface which may discourage use during surgery especially of the fairly bulky (5 cm long) probes. On the other hand, smaller probes (3 cm) have the disadvantage of providing a very confined field of view, making interpretation at times arduous.

2. Convex probes. This recently developed technology is proving highly successful in conventional ultrasound. Here the individual crystals of a multiple-crystal probe are given a convex arrangement so as to give a divergent ultrasound beam. As yet, however, their usefulness for intraoperative applications has still to be fully assessed.

3. Sectorial probes. These can be either mechanical or electronic. Mechanical probes – still the most common today – comprise one or more oscillating or rotating transducers. The image obtained is triangular or sectorial, the apex of the triangle being the point nearest the transducer. Although the much smaller contact surface of the sectorial probe is an advantage over the linear probe, sectorial probes give only poor focussing of superficial layers. However, much better results are now being seen with the new generation of electronic sectorial probes where a divergent beam is produced by exciting the many small transducers making up the probe at different intervals or in a staggered fashion. 'Annular array' transducers are the latest addition to this group of sectorial probes. Here the individual crystals are arranged concentrically and have different focussing points [3].

Doppler-ultrasound

With this new technique venous and arterial vascular flows can be assessed directly and non-invasively [1, 4].

The technique exploits the Doppler effect whereby echoes reflecting off a moving object have a different frequency from the incident ultrasound wave. This difference is a function of speed and is expressed as a particular mathematical equation = $F_D = \frac{2F_0 V C \alpha}{C}$, where F_D is the Doppler frequency (difference between the frequency of the incident and the reflected ultrasound waves), F_0 is the frequency of the incident ultrasound wave, C is the speed of ultrasound in soft tissues, α is the angle of incidence and V the velocity of the medium reflecting the ultrasound beam. Thus if the frequency variations are known, flow velocity can be calculated. Furthermore the frequency variations can be represented as acoustic signals audible to the human ear. These frequencies will vary positively (Fig. 1.2) or negatively depending on whether blood flow is towards or away from the transducer and will be displayed accordingly either above or below the baseline on the screen.

Duplex-ultrasound is the combination of the Doppler technique with real-time ultrasound. By means of real-time ultrasound the operator visualizes the vessel, which enables him to correctly place the 'sample volume' over the lumen to pick up the frequency variations. Sample volume is the region of the ultrasound beam sensitive to the presence of Doppler-shifted echoes. The axial position and extent of the sample volume are under operator control. Both vessel diameter and cross-sectional surface area are easily calculated with real-time ultrasound; once average flow velocity has been calculated, average output in ml/min. can be determined for the vessel in that particular point. Attention has to be paid, however, to errors produced by wrong measurement of the angle of incidence, particularly in tortuous vessels as this may significantly affect the calculation of flow velocity. The most suitable angles for this kind of measurement are between 30 and 60. Over this limit flow velocity cannot be correctly determined.

Special computer software has now been developed for ultrasound equip-

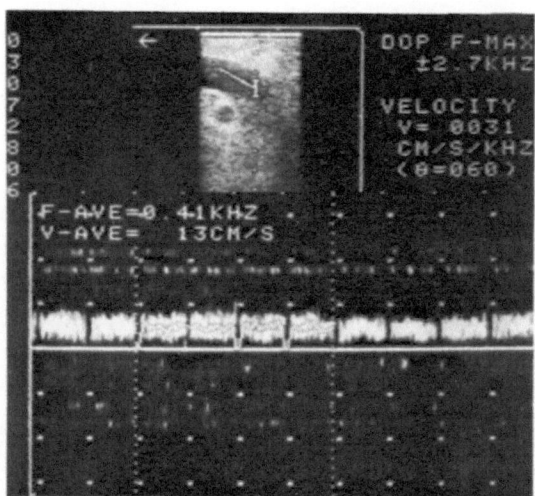

Figure 1.2. Intraoperative Duplex investigation of the splenic vein. Top: 2-D image of the splenic vein with the sample volume in vessel. Note the angle of incidence of the ultrasound beam to the main axis of the vessel. Below: spectral analysis of the frequency variations. Computer software program provide automatic calculation of avarage blood flow velocity (= 13 cm/ sec).

ment that enables all available probes – including intraoperative probes – to carry out Doppler flow investigation. The future potential of this new method is therefore readily appreciable.

References

1. Burns P., Joffe C.: *Quantitative flow measurements with Doppler ultrasound: techniques, accuracy and limitations.* Radiol. Clin. N. America, 23: 64, 1985.
2. Carlsen E. N.: *Ultrasonic physics for the physician: a brief review.* J. Clin. Ultrasound. 3: 69, 1975.
3. Carpenter D. A.: *Ultrasonic transducer in 'New Techniques and instrumentation in ultrasonography',* Walls P. N. T. and Zidkin M. C. – Eds. Churchill Livingston, New York, pp. 69–84, 1980.
4. Gill R.: *Measurement of the blood flow by ultrasound: accuracy and sources of error.* Ultrasound Med. Biol. II: 625–641, 1985.
5. Rose J. L., Goldberg B.B.: *Basic Physics in diagnostic ultrasound.* J. Wiley, New York, 1979.
6. Taylor K. J. W.: *Introduction to basic principles in 'Manual of Ultrasonography'.* Taylor K. J. W., Jacobson P., Talmont C. A., Winters R. Eds. Churchill Livingstone, New York, pp. 1–21, 1980.
7. Wells P. N. T.: *Real time scanning system, in 'New Techniques and instrumentation in Ultrasonography'.* Wells P. N. T. and Ziskin M. C. Eds. Churchill Livingstone, New York, pp. 69–84, 1980.

Chapter 2: Intra-operative ultrasonography: instrumentation and exploration technique

The first tentative applications of ultrasound during surgery made use of 'A mode' type equipment [5, 9, 11, 14] which merely represented the echoes as peaks or spikes of differing amplitude. Today's real-time machines not only afford immediate, dynamic imaging but have largely overcome problems related to probe-tissue contact and handling.

Intraoperative *ultrasonographic equipment* does not differ from other types of ultrasound apparatus. However, it should be compact, easy to handle and coupled to a suitably large monitor to enable the surgeon – about a meter away – to see comfortably. Controls should be easy and simple to enable trouble-free adjustment of luminosity, contrast and gain by medical staff. These are the only specific requirements for operative applications. The authors have experience with Toshiba SAL 32 and SAL 35 equipment and more recently, especially for Doppler applications, with the Ansaldo-Hitachi AU450.

Probes should be small, easily sterilized and, no less important, have a sufficient length of flex or cable (about 2 meters). Ultrasound frequency is high – from 5 to 10 MHz. The 5 MHz probe is a good compromise between resolution power and maximal depth of exploration (12 cm) and is particularly indicated in liver surgery [1, 3, 7, 8]. Higher frequencies – 7.5 or even on occasion 10 MHz – are for use in biliary and pancreatic [10, 12, 15] or endocrine gland [4] surgery where the tissue under observation is very thin. Sectorial probes may be advisable during biliary tract-pancreatic surgery on account of the small surface area that need come into contact with tissue [10, 12, 15]. In our experience, however, linear probes have proved suitable not only in liver but also in biliary tract and pancreatic surgery: images are more immediate and more readily understandable to the surgeon than the somewhat distorted image produced by the convex sectorial probe.

Various *types of probes* suitable for abdominal exploration (Table 2.1) are available on the market. 'T' shaped probes with the field of view on the side of the horizontal bar of the T, are used on the liver. In this way the probe can be held comfortably in the surgeon's palm and easily moved over the whole anterior face of the liver from the dome to the hepatic margin. Exploration is particularly easy in the case of right sub-costal laparotomy. 'T' shaped probes have a wide field of view, from 5 to 7 cm. The resultant imaging of the whole parenchyma aids in establishing the confines between lesions and surrounding vascular structures.

Smaller elements, known as 'razor probes' (Toshiba 'micro 10 B') have a narrower field of view (3 cm) and thus do not provide an overall picture,

Table 2.1. Instrumentation for intra-operative ultrasonography

	Sigel [15]	Lane	Jakimowicz [10]	Bismuth [1]	Gozzetti
Equipment	High Stoy	Xenotec	Philips	Aloka CGR	Toshiba
Transducer	Sector	Sector	Sector (small parts)	Linear (7 cm)	Linear (5 or 3 cm)
Frequency	7.5–10	10	5–7.5	5	5
Sector angle (degrees)	18	30–60			
Field of view (depth in mm)	60		40–110	120	120
Applications	Biliary tree Pancreas	Biliary tree Pancreas	Biliary tree Pancreas	Liver Biliary tree	Liver Biliary tree Pancreas

making topographic studies more arduous. However, they are very compact and can be used in the case of small incision laparotomy.

There are other versions of the 'T' probe, with the field of view on the top of the horizontal bar of the T. Finally there is the 'infradigital' or 'I' shaped probe (Fig. 2.1) that can also be employed in biliary tract, pancreatic, vascular or renal surgery.

The probe is placed directly on the organ to be investigated and moved by the surgeon. No coupling gels are required since the peritoneal fluid itself ensures excellent probe-tissue contact. The probe should be moved slowly and smoothly. The relations between lesion mass and surrounding structures are best demonstrated by 3-D assessment; this can be achieved by moving the probe lengthwise, obliquely and then longitudinally. The ultrasound images can then be recorded on a videotape or photographed on film (Polaroid 667). Usually intraoperative ultrasound study can be completed in 5–10 minutes.

In intraoperative ultrasonography the area to be examined is usually in direct contact with the probe. While this offers the advantage of allowing the use of higher frequencies with consequent better axial resolution, focussing is jeopardized. In fact in the operative setting, focussing the first few centimeters

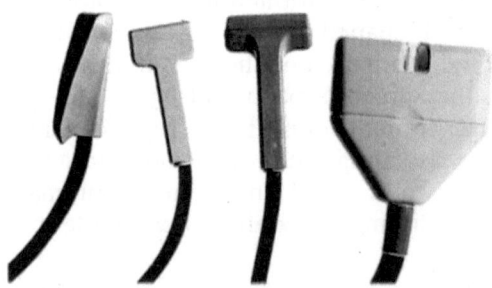

Figure 2.1. Probes for intraoperative ultrasound.

of the ultrasound beam is always a difficult business. If the area under study is in direct contact with the probe, an artefact in the form of a hyperechoic band is formed (also known as the 'bang effect') and no meaningful assessment can be made. Nor is this drawback overcome by automatic electronic focussing equipment.

As a countermeasure, some probes come with a frontal pad filled with liquid *(water path)* or oil. This puts a few centimeters between the point of emission and the tissue so as to bring the latter within the focal zone. This solution has been adopted especially for sectorial probes.

Recently, however, a new synthetic material has been made available [6]. Manufactured by 3M by combining a synthetic polymer with an inert oil, kitecko – as this material is called – is elastic, pliable and comes in various sizes. Kitecko has acoustic properties similar to water in that it does not produce any echo and therefore does not alter the formation of the under-lying ultrasound images. Placing kitecko between probe and tissue surface goes some way to solving the problem of focussing superficial tissue strata and adapting the probe to an irregular organ surface. Moreover the kitecko can be wrapped in a sterile adhesive cloth (Steril-Drape, 3M) which allows repeated sterilization (Fig. 2.2). Another way of overcoming the bang effect is to keep the operative field (and probe) flooded with saline while holding the

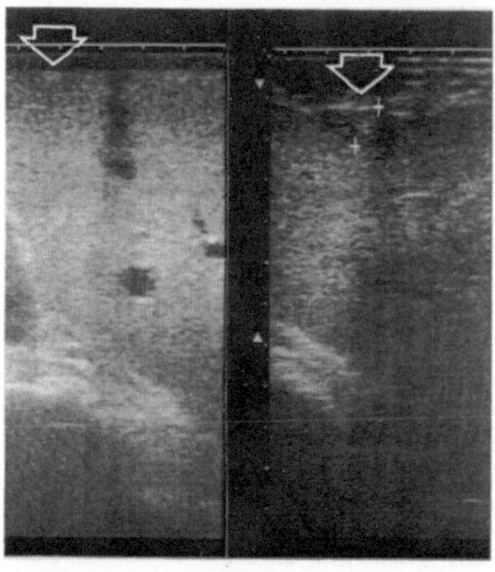 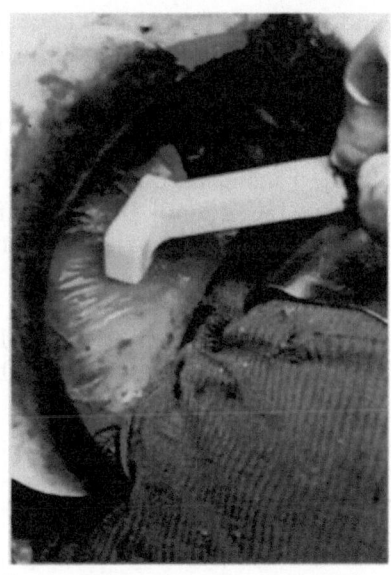

A   B   C

Figure 2.2.
A) Scan carried out with the probe touching the organ surface; the subcapsular lesion indicated by the arrow (metastasis of primary colon carcinoma) is only just visible.
B) Using a gel pad wrapped in adhesive sterile drape, the same lesion is now clearly visible as a 1 cm thick ultrasound band.
C) A *kitecko pad* wrapped in Steril drape.

probe about 1–2 cm away from the tissue surface. Others use thin plastic balloons filled with saline [1, 3]. The drawback here, however, is that the balloon tends to slip out from between probe and tissue surface.

Probe sterilization can be with gas or germicide solutions. Ethylene oxide is the surest method since it kills germs, spores and viruses. However steriliza-tion takes more than 24 hours of total immersion which, of course, consider-ably curtails instrument usage. Formalin vapor sterilization is faster, the probe being ready for re-use after 5–6 hours. For gas sterilization the probe must be wrapped in a double layer of plastic sheeting: after sterilization the whole package can be placed, ready for use, on the operating table. It is important to wrap plastic or alluminium foil around the connection between probe and flex to prevent transducer oxydation. The fastest sterilization procedure is total immersion of both probe and cable in Ibitane or Cidex germicide solu-tion, although complete virus kill is probably not achieved. Another viable method is to use the probe enclosed in a sterile plastic bag [10]. The probe face must first be covered with coupling gel and care must be taken to avoid folds in the plastic or trapped air bubbles which could generate artefacts. Furthermore this plastic covering should continue some way up the flex.

Lesions detected during operative scan can be biopsied under ultrasound guidance. For this purpose special probes have been developed with a central canal for the biopsy needle. The lesion is located and *biopsy* carried out under the continuous guidance of real-time ultrasound. These *'bored probes'* (Fig. 2.1), however, provide an image of inferior quality on account of the central blind spot created by the needle canal. Visualising the needle is itself invariably a problem since it lies parallel to the ultrasound beam. This has led to the recent development of *lateral adapters* for linear probes where the needle runs at an oblique angle to the beam. In some models this angle is variable [30, 45, 60]. In this way most of the needle lies across the path of the ultrasound waves and thus returns an echo which is then displayed on the screen (Fig. 2.3).

Core biopsy needles are used (Surecut, Trucut), with an external diameter ranging from 0.6 mm (23 G) to 1.2 mm (18 G), to take a specimen for histo-logical examination or a Chiba (0.7 mm, 22 G) needle when only a cytological study is required.

References

1. Bismuth H., Castaing D.: *Echographie pré-opératoire du foie et des vois biliaires*. Flam-marion Med. Sci. Paris, 1984.
2. Boldrini G., De Gaetano A. M.: *Ecografia intra-operatoria in chirurgia generale*. Mazza-pese Ed. (Roma) 1986.
3. Castaing D., Kunstlinger F., Habib N., Bismuth H.: *Intraoperative ultrasonographic study of the liver*. Am. J. Surg. 149. 676–682, 1985.
4. Chapuis Y., Hermigon A., Plainfosse M. C., Bonnette P.: *Exemples d'application de l'ultra-sonographie temps réel pré-opératoire en chirurgie endocrinienne*. Chirurgie 110: 97–104, 1984.

13

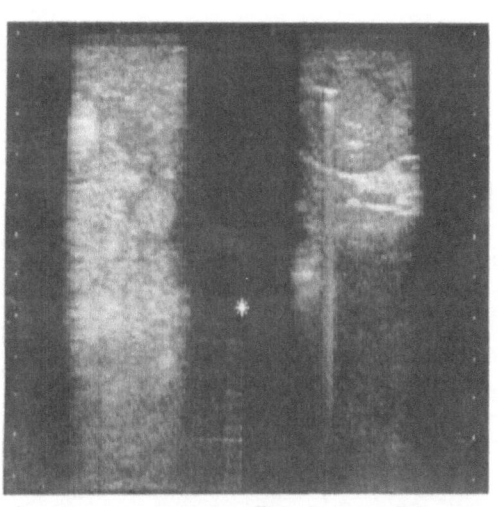 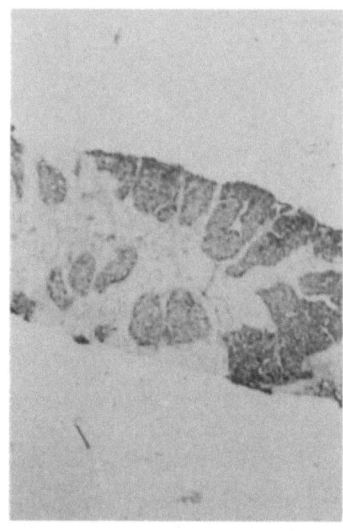

A   **B**   C

Figure 2.3. Needle biopsy guided by ultrasonography.
A) Massive right lateral hepatocarcinoma in cirrhotic liver.
B) Operative ultrasound evidences a non-palpable nodule of 1.5 cm in the 3rd segment. The highly echo-dense needle is clearly visible coursing obliquely toward the lesion. Biopsy needles can remove a tissue core for histological examination (C).

5. Eiseman B., Greenlaw R. H., Gallagher J. G.: *Localization of common duct stones by ultrasound.* Arch. Surg. 91: 195–199, 1965.
6. Fornage B. D., Touche D. H., Rifkin M. D.: *Small-parts real time sonography: a new weterpath.* T. Ultrasound Med. 3: 355–357, 1984.
7. Gozzetti G., Mazziotti A., Bolondi L., Cavallari A., Casanova P., Grigioni V., Bellusci R., Villanacci V., Labò G.: *Intraoperative ultrasonography in surgery for liver tumors.* Surgery 99: 523–529, 1986.
8. Gozzetti G., Mazziotti A., Bolondi L., Cavallari A., Casanova P.: *L'ecografia intraoperatoria in chirurgia addominale.* Chirurgia Epatobiliare, 1986.
9. Hayaski S., Wagai T., Miyazawa R.: *Ultrasonic diagnosis of breast tumor and cholelitiasis.* West J. Surg. Obstet Gynecol. 70: 34–36, 1962.
10. Jakimowicz J. J., Carol E. J., Jurgens P.: *The preoperative use of real-time B-mode ultrasound imaging in biliary and pancreatic surgery.* Dig. Surg. 1: 55–60, 1984.
11. Knight P. R., Newell J. A.: *Operative use of ultrasonic in cholelithiasis.* Lancet I: 1023–1025, 1963.
12. Lane R. J., Glazer G.: *Intraoperative B-mode ultrasound scanning of the extrahepatic biliary system and pancreas.* Lancet 334, 1980.
13. Makuuchi M.: *Abdominal Intraoperative Ultrasonography.* Igaku-Shoin Ed. (Tokyo) 1987.
14. Schlebel J.O., Diggdon P., Cuellar J.: *The use of ultrasound for localizing renal calculi.* J. Urol. 86: 367–369, 1961.
15. Sigel B.: *Operative ultrasonography.* Lea and Fabinger, Philadelphia, 1982.

Chapter 3: Ultrasound terminology

Over the years a special terminology has developed to define the alterations evidenced by ultrasound and a basic grounding in this is essential for an understanding of ultrasonography.

As already described, ultrasound images are created by juxtaposing the echoes formed as the ultrasound beam passes through tissue – each echo being a spot of light on the screen whose luminosity varies according to a special 'grey scale'.

Essentially, there are specular echoes, which are returned by the large interfaces dividing two contiguous organs, and scattered echoes, characteristic of the internal matrix of the various organs. This configuration of echoes, be it indicative of normal or pathological tissue, is commonly termed *'echo pattern'*. The echopattern of a given tissue may be homogeneously echogenic, anechoic, complex or mixed, hypoechoic, hyperechoic or inhomogeneous.

Homogeneous echogenic echopattern

The appearance is of a compact mesh of fine scattered echoes of uniform distribution and amplitude. Hollow structures such as vessels or ducts stand out clearly on account of their different acoustic impedance. Typical of this homogeneous echogenicity are the parenchyma of healthy tissues such as the liver (Fig. 3.1), spleen, pancreas, thyroid and testis.

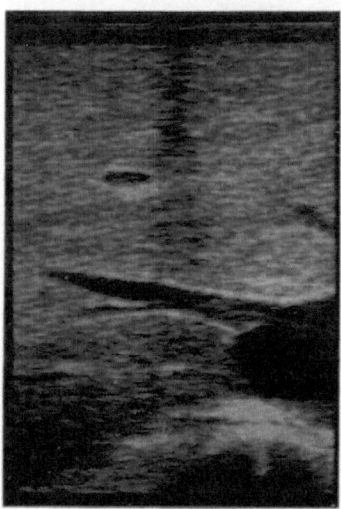

Figure 3.1. Normal liver. The homogeneous echoic echostructure of the parenchyma is interrupted by anechoic channels representing the intra-hepatic vessels (scan of the right lobe of the liver).

16

Anechoic echopattern

Characterized by a total absence of echoes even at high gain setting and generally accompanied by *'posterior wall enhancement'* (Fig. 3.2), which is the effect produced when the ultrasound beam undergoes no attenuation on

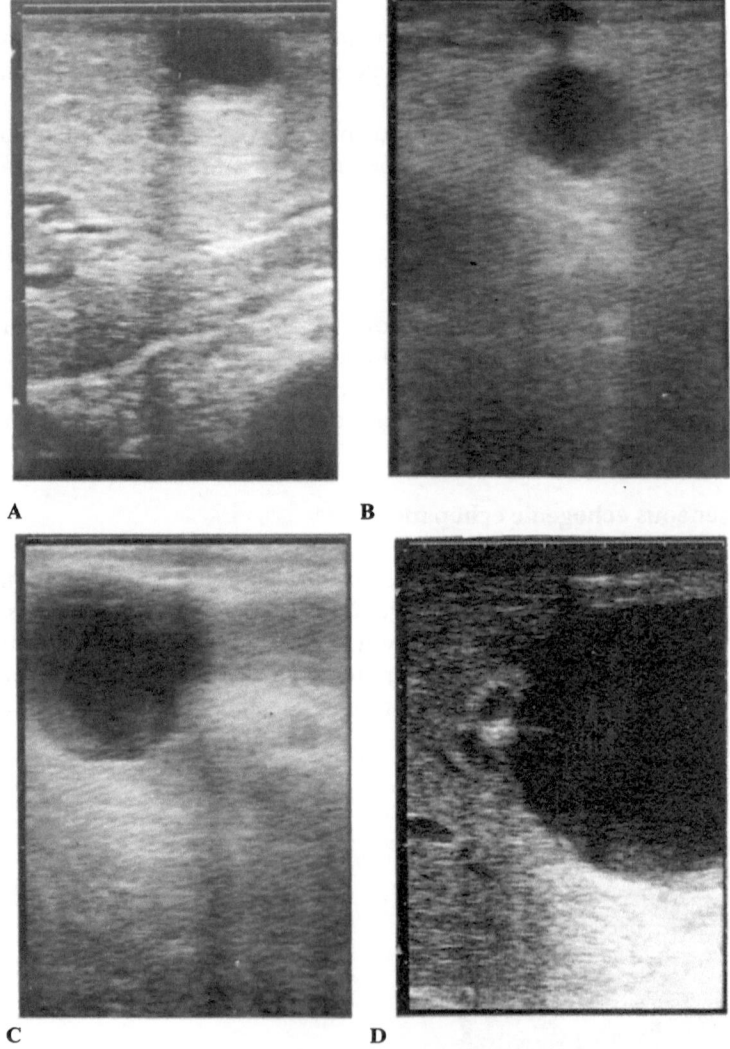

A   B

C   D

Figure 3.2. Fluid-filled cysts with characteristic anechoic appearance and posterior wall enhancement.
A, B) Serous cysts in the liver.
C) Cysts of the upper pole of the kidney.
D) Huge serous cyst of the liver with evident posterior wall enhancement. At intraoperative ultrasound neither walls nor septa are evidenced. The content of the cyst is homogeneous. These features differentiate the serous from the hydatid cyst.

passing through bodily structures that generate no echoes (as in the case of most fluids such as bile, blood, urine, amniotic fluid). Echo-free areas may also be indicative of pathology: cysts and uncomplicated pseudocysts, pouch collections of fluids and effusions into serous cavities, all return no echoes.

Mixed or complex echopatterns

Here echo-free or anechoic zones alternate with areas full of echoes of varying size and distribution. Usually transmission of the ultrasound beam through the echo-spared zones into deeper tissue is good and attenuation only very slight. Examples of complex echopattern masses are echinococcus cysts with associated daughter cysts (Fig. 3.3), cysts or pseudocysts containing large amounts of debris from necrosis, hemorrhage or infection, hematomas, cystomas and cystoadenocarcinomas and aneurysms with parietal thrombi. Moreover some 'impure' fluids may also generate a complex echopattern: purulent collections (Fig. 3.4), the content of the stomach after a meal, etc.

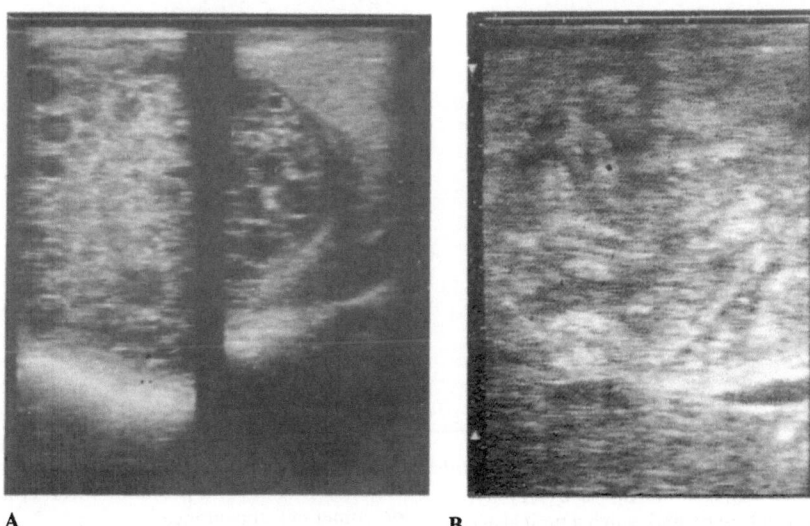

A   B

Figure 3.3.
A) *Hydatid cyst of the liver* with typical complex echostructure (mixed solid and fluid) due to numerous daughter cysts (small rounded anechoic lacunae).
B) *Hydatid cyst of the liver* with a complex echopattern due to the presence of wavy echoic structures which represent membranes and dead cysts immersed in a small amount of fluid.

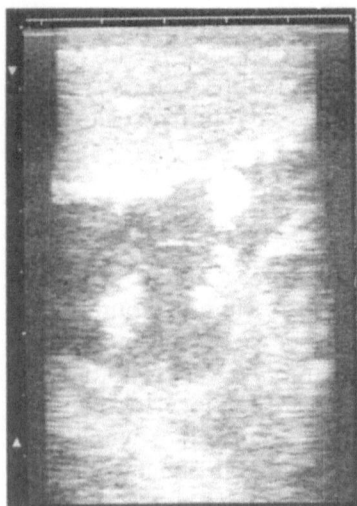

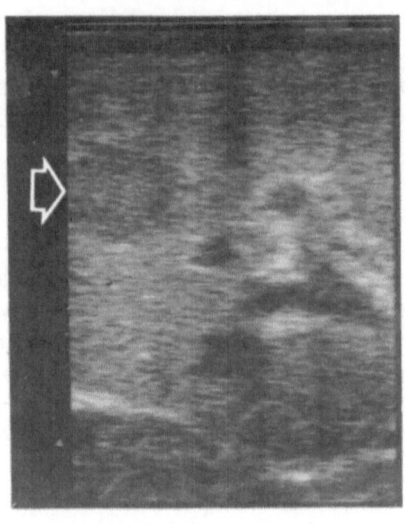

Figure 3.4. Hepatic abscess. Inhomogeneous fluid collection in segment 7. The irregular echogenic pattern is due to cellular debris and fibrin deposits.

Figure 3.5. *Small (1.5 cm) hypoechoic hepatocarcinoma* (arrow).

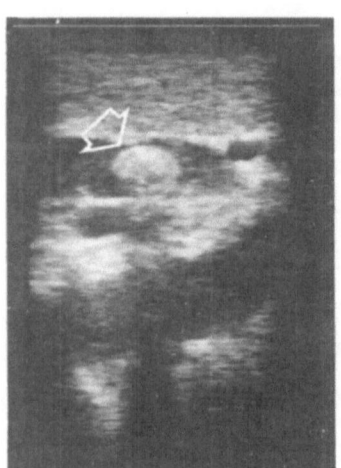

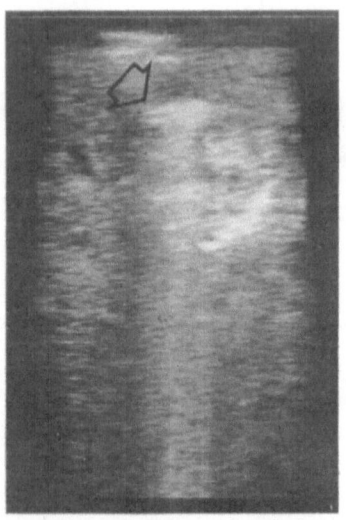

Figure 3.6. *Stone* (arrow) *of the common bile duct.* The stone shows up as a very hyperechoic structure behind which a typical acoustic shadow cone is observed.

Figure 3.7. *Aerobilia* (arrow): typical hyperechoic structure with posterior reverberation or 'comet tail' appearance.

Hypoechoic echopattern

A hypoechoic image is returned when only few interfaces are present. The echoes returned, however, are of low amplitude, tending to increase if the gain setting is increased. Attenuation is slight and consequently the ultrasound beam is carried into deep-lying tissue. However the phenomenon of posterior wall enhancement is not normally seen. This echopattern is typical of normal soft tissue like muscle and lymph nodes whose echogenicity is much lower that of the liver, spleen etc., or certain pathological tissue: acute inflammation of the parenchyma (eg. acute edematous pancreatitis); some types of intra-parenchymal tumor (small hepatocarcinomas) (Fig. 3.5), adenopathies, retro-peritoneal tumors (cancer of the pancreas).

Hyperechoic echopattern

The appearance is characterized by multiple high level echoes even at low gain. Depending on their architecture or constituent elements, hyperechoic structures give rise to *'acoustic shadows'* or *'reverberations'*.

In the first case (Fig. 3.6), an echo-free band is visible behind the hyper-echoic formation. This is due to the ultrasound beam being completely absorbed. Reverberation (Fig. 3.7) is caused by spurious echoes being formed

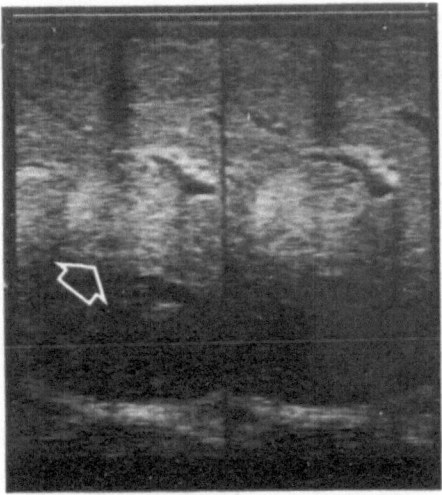 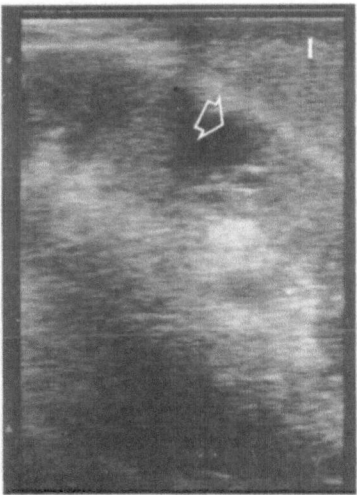

Figure 3.8. Hepatic angioma clearly showing hyperechoic nodules (arrow).

Figure 3.9. Right kidney, with small, 1 cm cyst in the cortex (arrow). The kidney has a prevalently irregular appearance, the cortex appearing evenly echogenic like the liver lying above (1), while the renal sinus is hyperechoic due to the presence of fat, connective tissue, vessels and lymphatic glands.

20

between the transducer and hyperechoic structure. Reverberations occur when interfaces of very different acoustic impedance are located near the transducer (eg. soft tissue/bone or soft tissue/gas interfaces).

Hyperechoic structures comprise both normal human parts: bone, cartilage, lung, gas in the alimentary canal, or pathological tissue: stones, calcification, scar tissue, certain scirrhous and infiltrating neoplasms. Some parenchymal lesions may also appear hyperechoic: hepatic angiomas (Fig. 3.8), some liver metastases, renal angiomyolipomas and thyroid adenomas. The echogenicity of the parenchyma is always enhanced by lipid infiltration (hepatic steatosis, sclerolipomatosis of the pancreas).

Inhomogeneous echopattern

Here hypoechoic areas alternate with hyperechoic zones indicating the presence of tissues of differing acoustic impedance. This is the case with normal organs such the breast, uterus and ovaries as well as the kidney where the cortex, medulla and renal sinus present very different echogenicity (Fig. 3.9). Among the pathological conditions presenting this uneven pattern are: 'target' or bull's-eye hepatic metastases (a central hyperechoic area surrounded by a hypoechoic halo); large hepatic angiomas (Fig. 3.10); some neoplasms with pockets of necrotic colliquation etc.

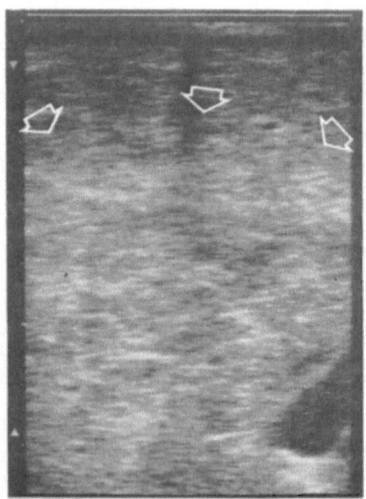

Figure 3.10. The typical irregular echopattern of a *cavernous hemangioma of the liver* (arrows).

Chapter 4: Intraoperative ultrasonography during liver surgery

Liver surgery is the main area of application for intraoperative ultrasonography.

The complex vascularization of the liver and the fact that there are no external landmarks on the liver surface indicating intrahepatic vessel location, along with the frequency of anatomic anomalies in the hepatic and Glisson branches, all pose considerable problems for the surgeon. The anatomical configuration of Couinaud [12, 13] and the surgical diagrams of Ton That Tung [62] are often of scant practical use especially in the case of a liver whose architecture has been severely distorted by cirrhosis or previous surgery.

Intraoperative ultrasound affords 'real time' investigation during surgery of the layout of the intrahepatic, hepatic and portal vessels, displaying any anatomical anomalies and showing intrahepatic vessel involvement in cystic or neoplastic disease. It provides a comprehensive segmental map for both normal as well as cirrhotic or otherwise damaged livers where structures have undergone alteration on account of tumor growth or previous operations.

Moreover, intraoperative ultrasound can pick up intrahepatic formations as small as 4–5 millimeters which would not be detected by CT Scan, angiography or even preoperative ultrasound. This is because intraoperative probes have a higher sound frequency than conventional abdominal transducers, and therefore resolution is increased. In fact intraoperative ultrasound is the ultimate diagnostic examination to detect liver tumors and as such can prompt more radical surgery where this is feasible, while excluding patients with disseminated intrahepatic disease who would derive no lasting benefits from surgery.

The advantages of intraoperative ultrasound are especially conspicuous in the case of cirrhotic livers where surgical exploration is more difficult and parenchymal tumors often fail to be detected on palpation. The increasingly wide use of intraoperative ultrasound during liver surgery has led to more accurate identification of size and location of tumors and their relationship with intrahepatic vascular structures and has enabled more radical but at the same time, more selective surgery [3, 7, 8, 10, 19, 21, 22, 27, 39, 40, 41, 42, 44, 55, 61, 63].

The technique of intraoperative echographic exploration of the liver

Both right subcostal laparotomy and midline incisions – to remove a tumor in the digestive tract – allow direct ultrasound exploration of the liver. Initially a 'micro' razor-blade or I-shaped probe can be used since both are easy to handle and give a complete view of the liver even through small-incision laparotomy. For ease of exploration, the falciform ligament should be incised to allow the probe to slip unhampered right along the anterior surface of the liver. Although coupling gel is not necessary, it does help to wet the probe periodically to ensure adherence to the liver capsule and consequent transmission of the ultrasound beam. Complete visualization of the liver can be achieved without preliminary sectioning of the triangular ligaments. Indeed these should be incised only once it has been ascertained that resection is feasible and in any case, only on the side of the involved hemisphere. In cirrhotic livers, incising the triangular ligament may prove difficult and there is the added risk of hemorrhage.

Shallow lesions lying directly under the capsule are either not detected at all or very poorly imaged by direct-contact ultrasound. To offset this, use a kitecko pad or cushion, wrapped in a sterile drape and take an oblique scan, or approach the liver from the inferior aspect.

Systematic exploration of the liver starts with the left lobe, first posteriorly (2nd segment) and then anteriorly (3rd segment). The portal peduncles are seen coursing in parallel across the left lobe; the lesser omentum appears as a clear hyperechoic strip and, under this, the caudate lobe overlying the inferior vena cava, which however can be seen to pulsate with respiration (Fig. 4.1). Below the caudate lobe, the aorta and celiac trunk are observed. From here the common hepatic artery can be followed as it veers to the right (the left on the display screen) (Fig. 4.1B).

Exploration of the right lobe should start at the hepatic dome. Once the hepatic veins have been located, shift the probe a few centimeters down the anterior face of the liver to visualize the bifurcation of the portal vein following its right and left branches. The individual segments of the right lobe are then explored up to the lateral aspect of the liver. At the top, the 7th segment adjoins the diaphragm and at the bottom, segment 6 rests on the right kidney and will move if compressed by the probe. This scan will also visualize the right adrenal gland (Fig. 4.2). If the probe is then laid longitudinally, the resultant sagittal scan will show the whole length of the retrohepathic vena cava as well as the caudate lobe.

Next comes the gall-bladder. The approach is transhepatic with the probe resting on the anterior face of the liver. This evidences the fundus of the gallbladder, the confluence of the right and left bile ducts and finally the hepatic peduncle where any anatomic anomalies will be evidenced, the most frequent being a right hepatic artery springing from the superior mesenteric artery which courses behind the portal vein.

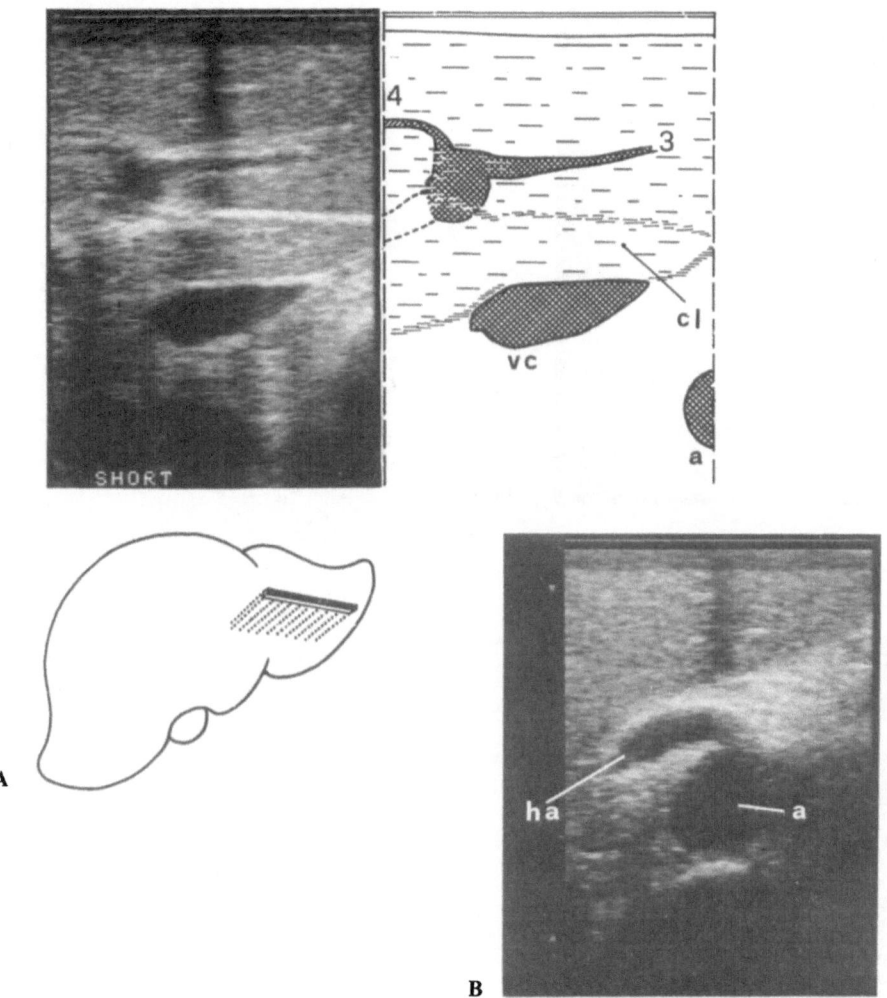

Figure 4.1.
A) *Transverse scan of the left lobe.* The recess of Rex is clearly visible. From here the left 'horn' goes to the 3rd segment and the right one to the 4th. Below, the gastrophepatic ligament appears as a very hyperechoic band separating segment 3 from the caudate lobe.
B) *Transverse scan of the 2nd segment.* The aorta (a) from which originate the celiac trunk and the hepatic artery (ha).

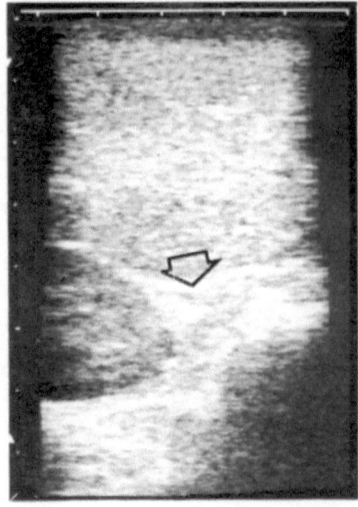

Figure 4.2. Oblique Scan of the 6th segment. Posterior to the liver, the upper pole of the right kidney is visible and above this, the typical 'Phrygian cap' pattern of the right adrenal (arrow).

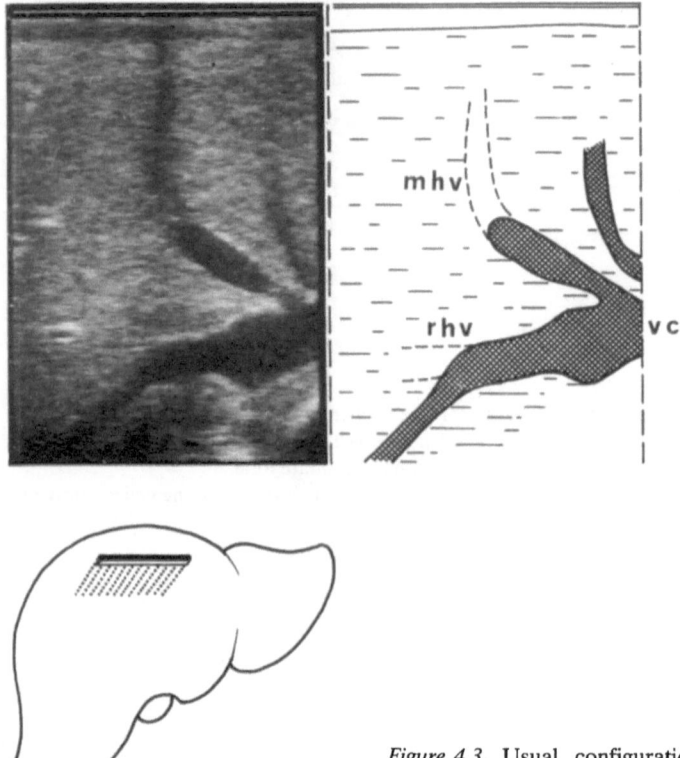

Figure 4.3. Usual configuration of hepatic veins draining into the vena cava.

Liver anatomy at ultrasound investigation

The oblique course of the *hepatic veins* towards the vena cava is generally well and easily visualized. With the exception of the juxta-caval portion of the right hepatic vein, the walls of these veins have no fibrous tissue sheath and therefore return no echoes. Blood flow through the vessels is clearly visible as fine echo turbulences. While the vessel lumen of non-cirrhotics can be easily compressed simply by pushing the probe against the liver surface, the veins of cirrhotic livers appear narrow and tortuous.

The point of entry of the hepatic veins into the vena cava is readily evidenced by placing the probe on the dome of the liver and tilting it slightly upwards. Modal configuration (i.e. the right hepatic vein having a single branch and the middle hepatic vein draining into the left hepatic vein) Fig. 4.3) is seen in approximately 2/3 of cases (37 of the 55 non-cirrhotic, apparently lesion-free livers examined during laparotomy). In these cases the hepatic vein of the 7th segment is clearly visible as it runs into the right hepatic vein just a few centimeters from the vena cava (Fig. 4.4). In about 1/4

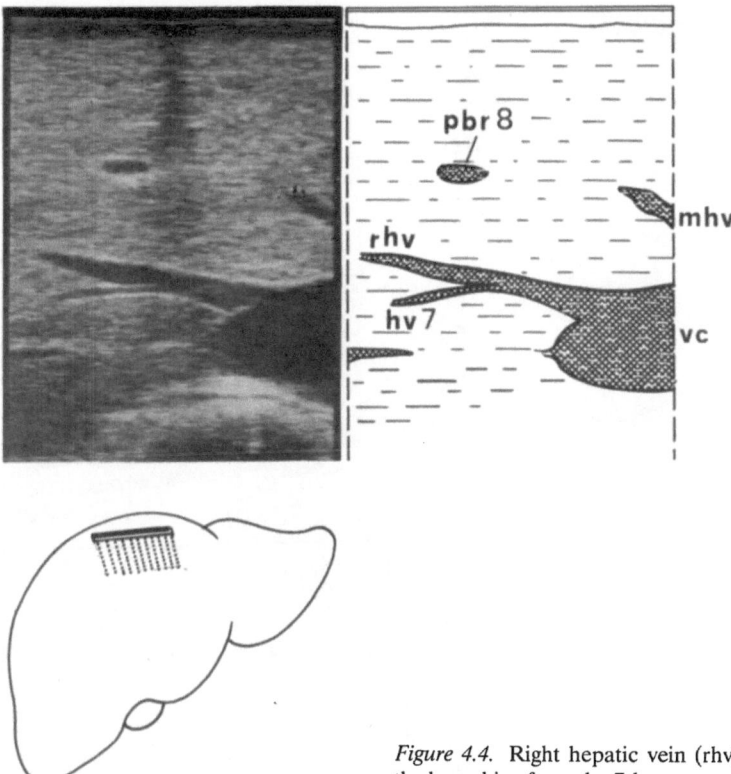

Figure 4.4. Right hepatic vein (rhv) draining the branching from the 7th segment (hv 7).

of cases, however, the middle hepatic vein drains into the vena cava separately (Fig. 4.5).

Other anomalies are:

- absence of the middle hepatic vein with, in its stead, many small veins draining into the vena cava at separate points (2 cases) (Fig. 4.5B);
- presence of a large vein in the 7th (1 case) or 6th segment (3 cases) entering the vena cava separately (Fig. 4.5);
- presence of a vein in the 8th segment flowing into the sagittal hepatic vein immediately adjacent to the vena cava (1 case) (Fig. 4.5D).

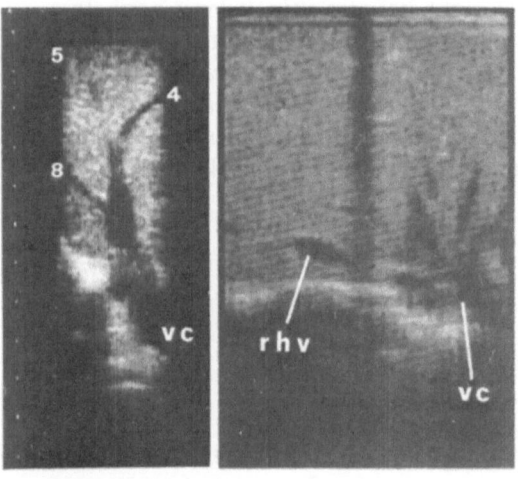

A   B

Figure 4.5. Anomalies of the hepatic veins.
A) The middle hepatic vein drains directly into the vena cava (vc). The collaterals from the 4th, 5th and 8th segments are also visible.
B) The middle hepatic vein is absent and in its stead there are several small veins.
C) The hypatic vein from the 7th segment drains separately into the vena cava.
D) Hepatic vein from the 8th segment.

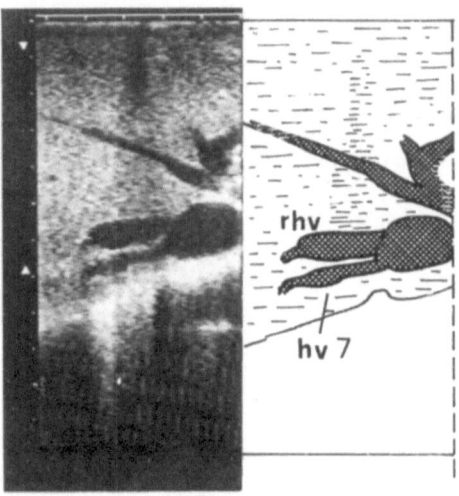

C

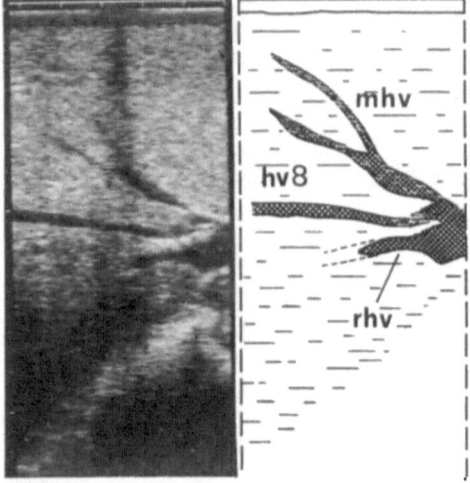

D

Portal Peduncles. The portal branches of the hepatic artery and bile ducts pass into the hilum of the liver sheathed in fibrous tissue, which accompanies them up to the peripheral ramifications. This tissue elicits a sharp hyperechoic halo which is visible right up to the point at which the portal peduncles ramify.

The different portal, arterial and biliary vessels can be distinguished only at the porta hepatis; after segmentary branching only the branches of the portal vein can be seen as sonolucent tubular bands.

Early on, the right branch of the portal vein divides into a paramedian branch coursing anteriorly and vertically, and a lateral branch running transversely. After about 2 cm the portal branch divides into an anterior branch to segment 5 and a posterior branch going to segment 8. The lateral branch – followed in transverse scans – divides into a long straight offshoot coursing to the 6th segment and to the periphery of the right liver and a posterior branch traveling upward to the 7th segment (Fig. 4.6). The tributaries to the right liver follow the plane of the right hepatic vein and can be visualized on cross sectional scan when the portal branches will present lying lengthwise and vice-versa. The left branch of the portal vein is longer and travels transversely. Above it lies the left branch of the bile duct. 2–3 smaller branches arise from the posterior aspect of the portal branch to drain the caudate lobe (Fig. 4.7). At the insertion of the falciform ligament the left portal branch becomes longitudinal and terminates in the recess of Rex. From here, a right branch arises to drain Riedel's lobe, a left going to the 3rd segment and – 1.5–2 cm from this – another branch runs transversely towards the 2nd segment (Fig. 4.1). Clear visualization of the intra-hepatic vessels allows accurate mapping of the liver segments since these are delimited laterally by the hepatic veins

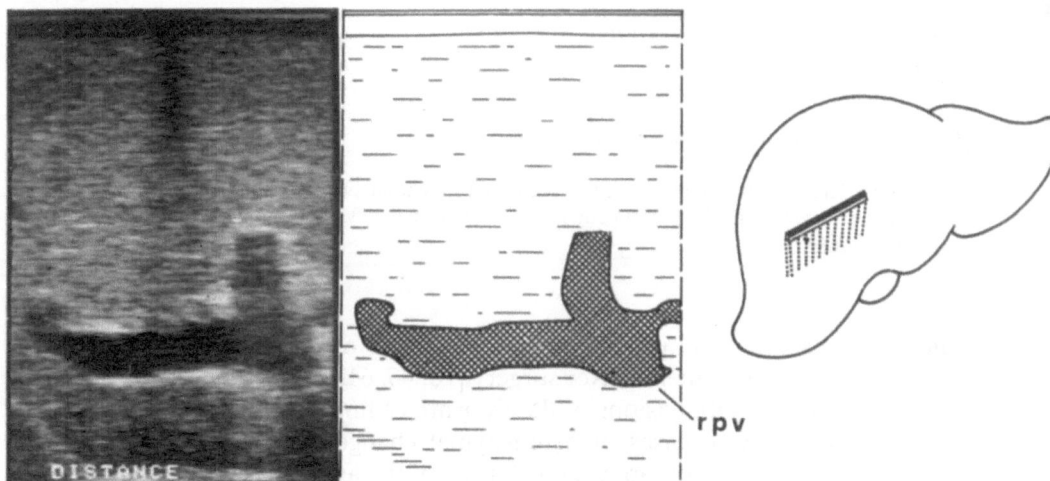

A

28

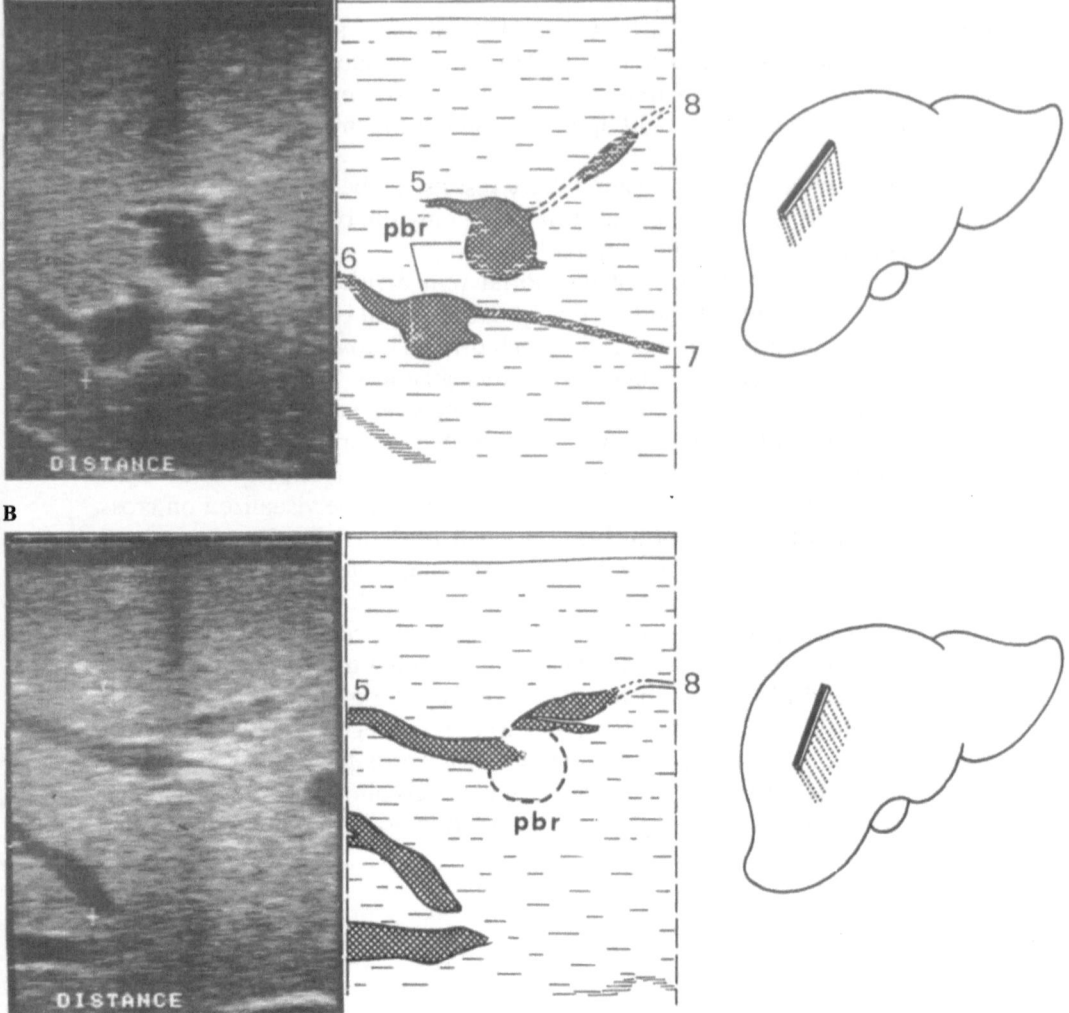

B

C

Figure 4.6. Portal vascularization of the right liver.
A) Scan across the hilum.
B) Oblique laterals can displaying the two sectorial branches in cross section.
C) Oblique scan showing the portal pedicles to segments 5 and 8.

and transversely by the protal peduncles. This is of considerable practical importance during segmental liver surgery [10, 47, 61, 63].

Often textbook subdivisions of the liver are of limited practical use to the surgeon, especially in cases of parenchymal changes induced by cirrhosis. Intraoperative ultrasonography allows study of the anatomy of the individual patient and as a result, can ensure more accurate segmental surgery.

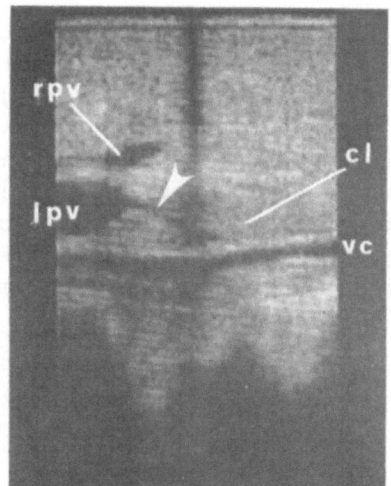

Figure 4.7. Longitudinal Scan showing the full length of the vena cava (vc) lying behind the liver, the right portal vein (rpv), left portal vein (lpv) and a branch (arrow) arising from the left portal vein and draining (the caudate lobe (cl).

Ultrasound appearances of liver tumors

Benign tumors

Angiomas. Small hemangiomata (less than 3 cm) appear as uniformly hyperechoic nodules with well defined margins and with no surrounding halo (Fig. 4.8). They are usually located near the inferior vena cava and hepatic veins and may cause posterior beam attenuation. This ultrasonic appearance is due to the angioma's abundant stromal tissue and vascular structures, comprising a complex web of capillaries. In other instances posterior enhancement may be present. On occasion however, small angiomas may appear hypo-or anechoic or echo-spared [20].

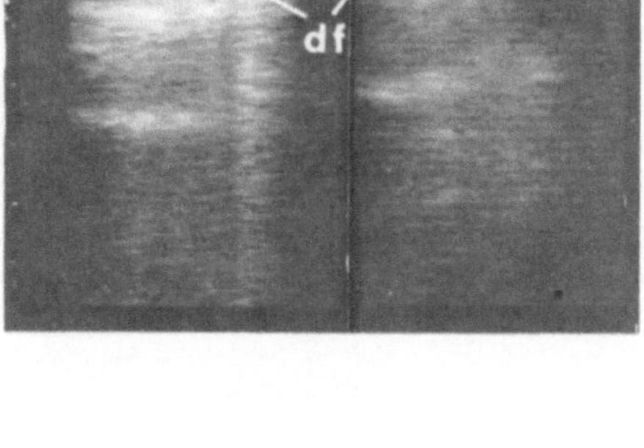

Figure 4.8. Small angiomas (an) in the 7th segment, adjacent to the diaphragm (df).

30

Large angiomas demonstrate an irregular pattern of echogenic and sono-lucent areas, with irregular and at times, poorly defined margins. The periph-eral halo is again absent (Fig. 4.9). This irregular appearance is due to throm-bosis and hemorrhage within these large formations as well as the presence of large blood lakes. While small angiomas present few diagnostic problems at ultrasound, huge angiomas can be difficult to differentiate from malignant neoplasms. At intraoperative ultrasound, however, pressure exerted by the probe on a large, characteristically compressible angioma, will cause a telling change in the ultrasound appearance (Fig. 4.10).

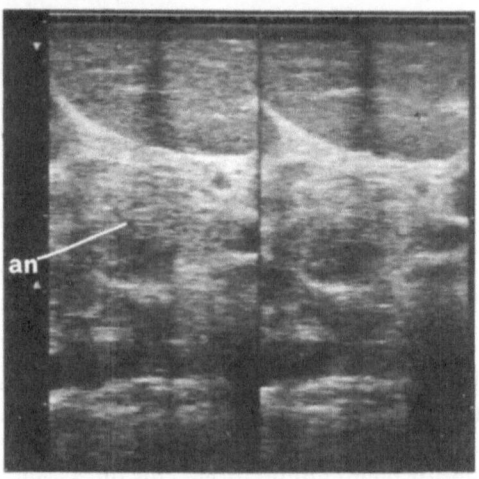

Figure 4.9. Cavernous angioma of segment 7). Pressure with the hand on the surface of the liver shows the lesion to be easily deformabled, becoming more echoic with the elimination of the blood lacunae and assuming a more flattened shape.

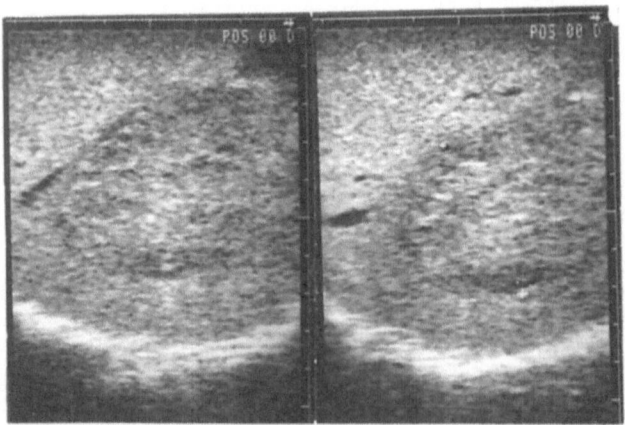

Figure 4.10. Cavernous angioma of the 7th segment. Pressing the hand on the liver surface will cause the lesion to deform and appear flatter and more echoic on account of blood volume reduction.

Adenomas. The ultrasonic appearance is of uniformly echoic or hypoechoic nodular formations of varying size, with possible anechoic areas indicating necrosis or hemorrhage.

Focal nodular hyperplasia. This appears as a solid, mainly uniform mass with only a few areas of different echogenicity. Massive lesions will been seen to compress and dislocate surrounding vessels (Fig. 4.11).

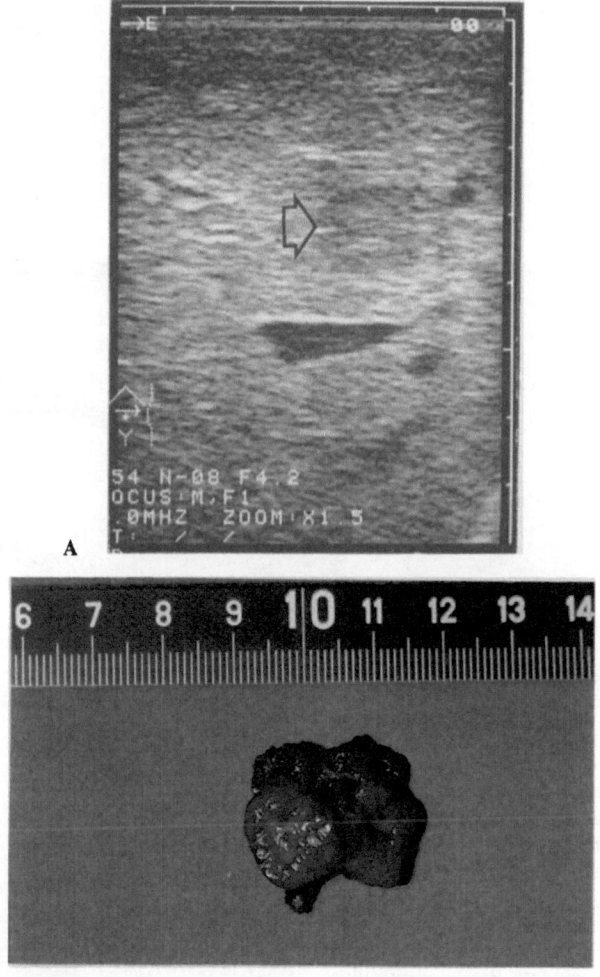

A

B

Figure 4.11. Focal nodular hyperplasia.
A) 50 year old patient with chronic liver disease. Routine ultrasonic examination showed a 2 cm hypoechoic nodule in the 4th segment. Although cytology was negative for malignant cells the patient underwent exploratory surgery on account of his pre-existing liver disease. Intra-operative ultrasound identified an unpalpable nodule of hypoechoic appearance and without a halo. This was removed with a wedge resection.
B) Histological examination confirmed the diagnosis of focal nodular hyperplasia.

32

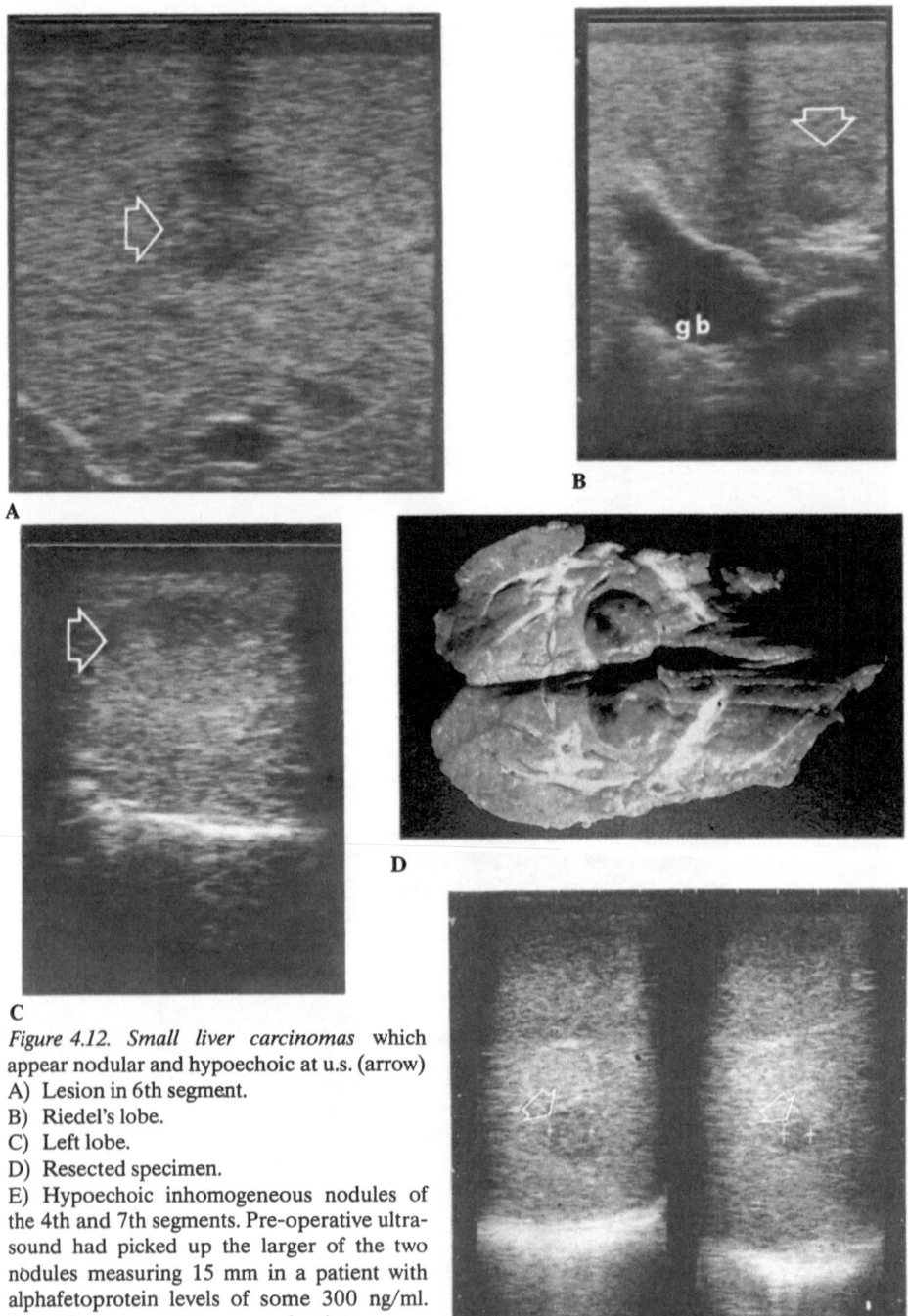

A

B

C

D

E

Figure 4.12. Small liver carcinomas which appear nodular and hypoechoic at u.s. (arrow)
A) Lesion in 6th segment.
B) Riedel's lobe.
C) Left lobe.
D) Resected specimen.
E) Hypoechoic inhomogeneous nodules of the 4th and 7th segments. Pre-operative ultra-sound had picked up the larger of the two nodules measuring 15 mm in a patient with alphafetoprotein levels of some 300 ng/ml. the patient was sent to surgery but intraopera-tive ultrasound revealed another locus in seg-ment 7 of 6 mm and hence hepatic resection was contraindicated.

Malignant tumors

Hepatocellular carcinomas have a variety of ultrasonic appearances, largely dependant on their size [14]. Small carcinomas are usually less echogenic than the surrounding parenchyma (Fig. 4.12). On occasion the echogenicity of both tumor and adjacent liver are very similar, making interpretation difficult. In such cases, a mass can be identified by moving the probe around to get a dynamic ultrasound picture of the adjacent parenchyma by way of contrast (Fig. 4.13). However, very extensive tumor masses appear so invasive that delineation of the neoplastic contours is no longer possible (Fig. 4.14).

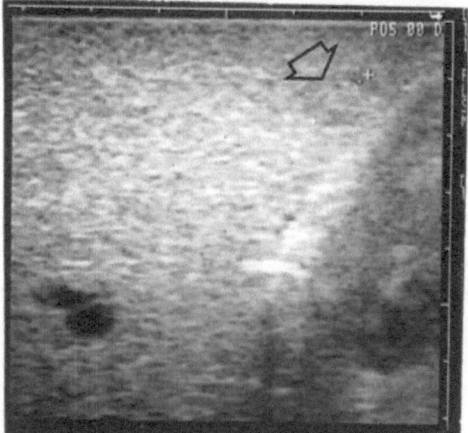

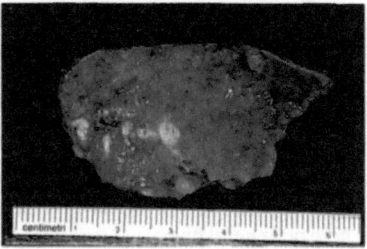

B

A

Figure 4.13.
A) *Small* (11 mm) *hepatocarcinoma* in cirrhotic liver with isoechoic echopattern (arrow).
B) Resected specimen.

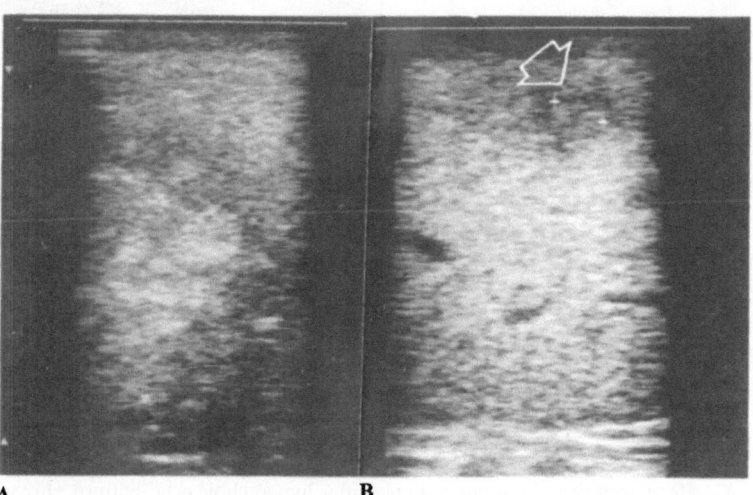

A   B

Figure 4.14. Large hepatocellular carcinoma of the right liver with irregular, ill defined contours (A). A daughter lesion can be seen 0.8 cm away on the 4th segment (B – arrow).

34

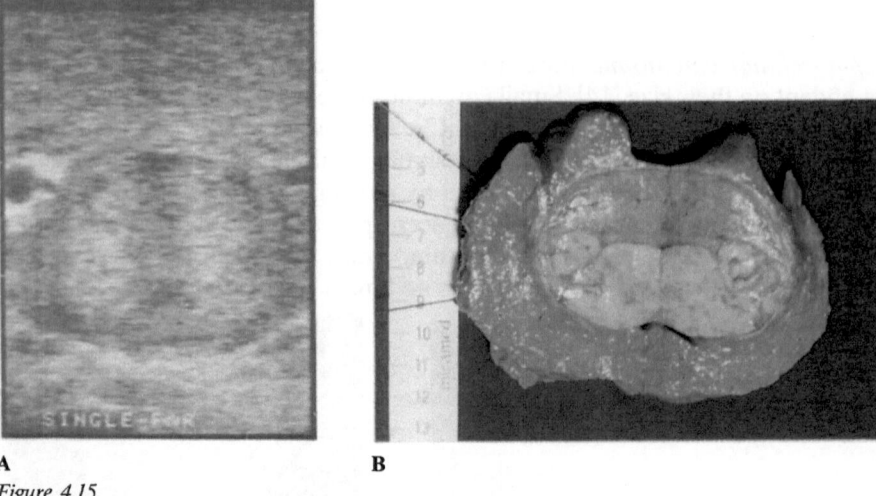

A   B

Figure 4.15.
A) *Hepatocellular carcinoma* of 3 cm diameter, presenting uniform echo-pattern with a hypo-echoic peripheral halo.
B) Resected piece. A thin capsule was found around the tumor.

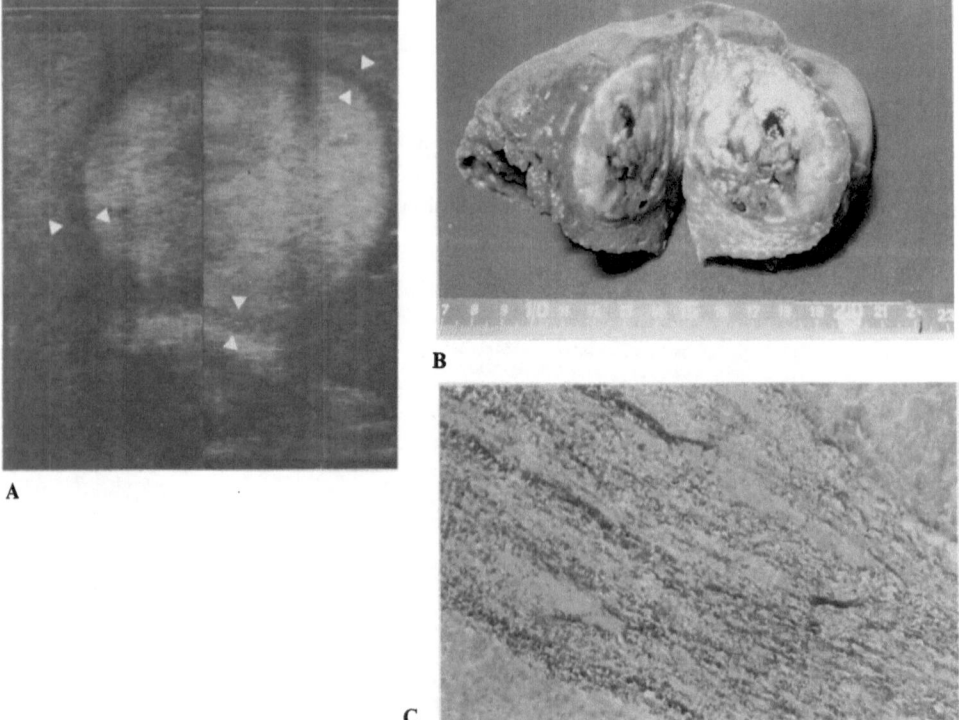

B

A

C

Figure 4.16. Hepatocellular carcinoma with irregular hyperechoic echo-pattern, surrounded by a visible hypoechoic halo (arrows), (A) which correspond to a capsule clearly visible on the sur-gical specimen (B) and at histologic examination (C).

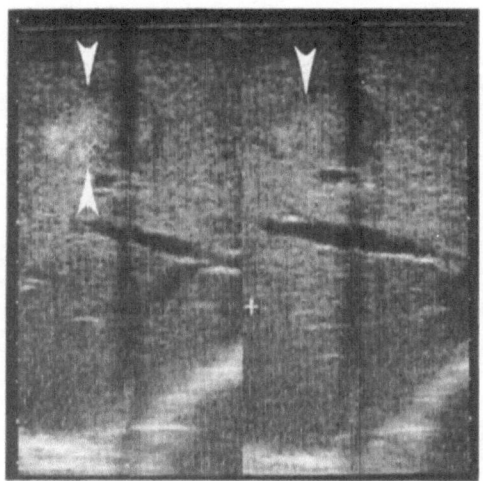 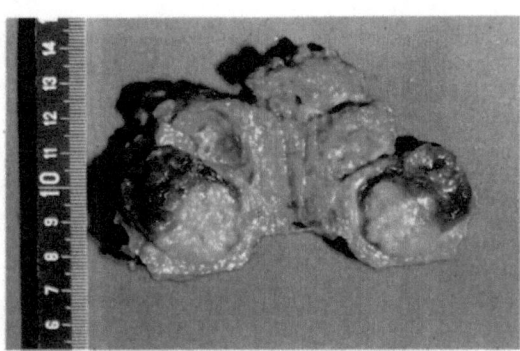

A   B

Figure 4.17. Small hepatocellular carcinoma in cirrhotic liver.
A) The hypoechoic halo is discontinuous on the right (left in figure – arrow) because of infiltration of the capsule by tumoral tissue.
B) The surgical specimen clearly shows the breach in the capsule made by the tumor.

Low level echoes usually correspond to tumors comprising neoplastic cells alone, while larger masses may also present mixed pattern echoes or even increased echogenicity due to the presence of fibrous tissue, hemorrhage or necrosis [14].

The finding of a thin hypoechoic peripheral halo (Figs. 4.15 and 4.16) is quite frequent in neoplasias of less than 5 cm and has been attributed to the presence of a fibrous capsule surrounding the tumor [56], which, moreover, is a favorable prognostic factor [21, 22, 60]. On occasion this peripheral halo may appear breached by the tumor spilling over into the surrounding tissue. In this case tumor contour is usually less sharp (Fig. 4.17). The characteristic halo is hardly ever seen in more voluminous neoplasias, which invariably present as irregularly marginated, hyperechoic or mixed-pattern masses.

Of considerable diagnostic and prognostic importance is the presence of *vascular infiltration*. This presents either as a sudden interruption of an intrahepatic vessel, the presence of dense echogenic material inside the lumen or as an ill-defined vessel wall profile. *Cholangiocarcinomas* appear as either hyperechoic or isoechoic lesions, as in liver metastases which in fact they resemble even macroscopically (Fig. 4.18).

Metastases. Liver metastases present a variety of appearances which sometimes may be seen in the same patient (Fig. 4.19). Most frequent are:
– single or multiple highly echogenic lesions;
– hypoechoic lesions with scattered areas of irregular echopattern within the mass;

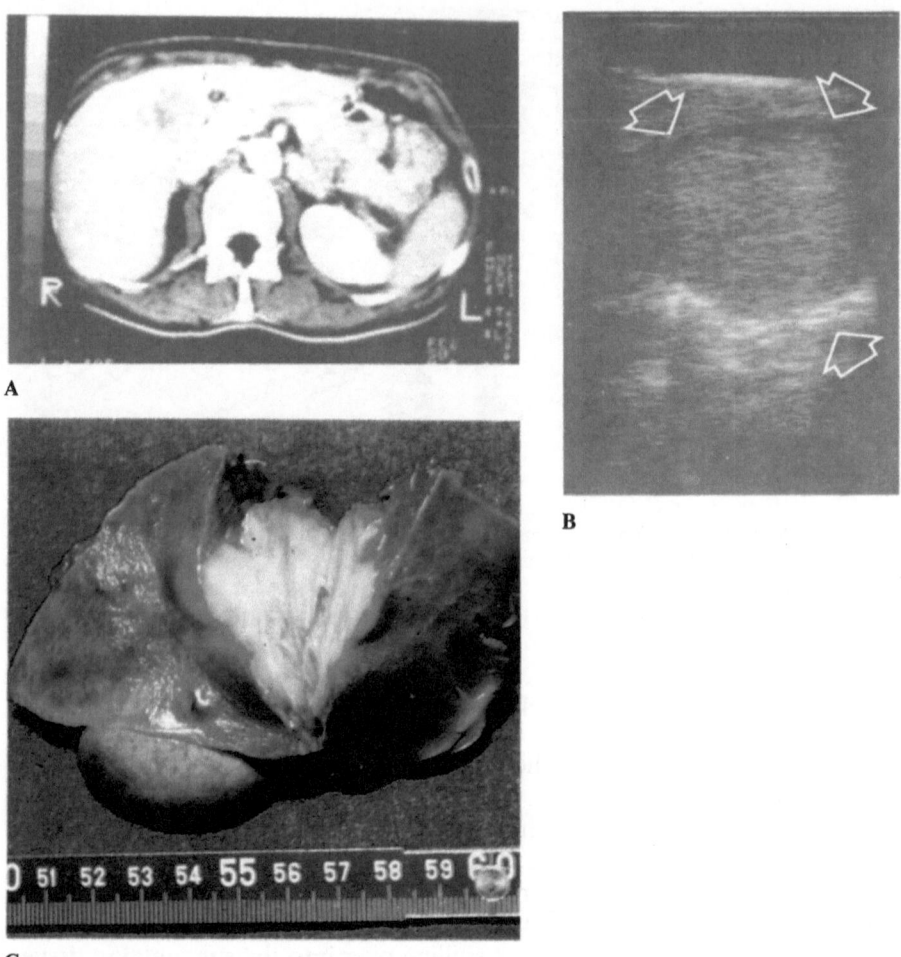

A

B

C

Figure 4.18. Cholangiocarcinoma in the 4th segment of the liver.
A) CT scan of the liver using contrast medium: low density lesion.
B) Uniformly echogenic lesion with sharply defined margins separating it from surrounding parenchyma (arrow). Examination carried out with kitecko gel pad.
C) Surgical piece following bisegmentectomy of 4–5.

– nodular 'bull's eye' lesions in which a central echogenic area is surrounded
  by a hypoechoic halo.
Correlation between ultrasound appearances and histologic metastatic type
has shown that hyperechoic masses tend as a rule to be metastases of colorectal carcinomas while hypoechoic patterns generally prove to be secondary forms of mesenchymal tumor [65]. Tumor vascularization has been correlated to echogenicity, with highly vascularized lesions appearing more echogenic than poorly vascularized masses [52].

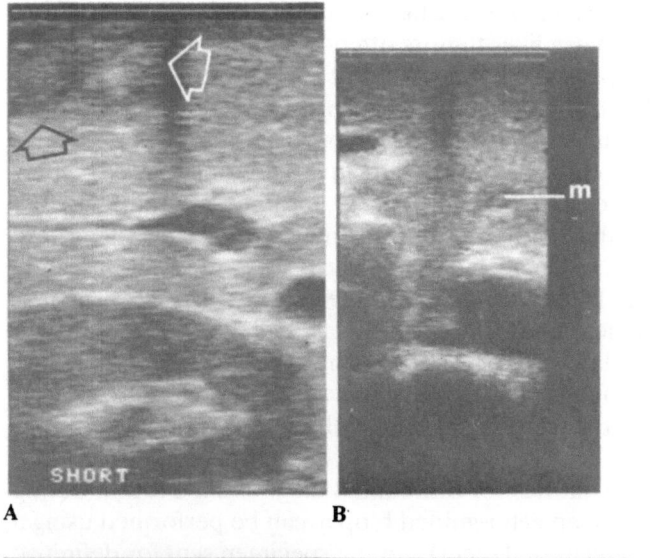

SHORT

A   B

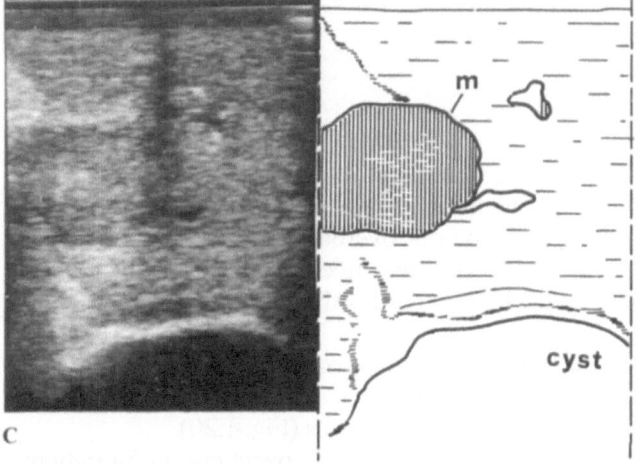

m

cyst

C

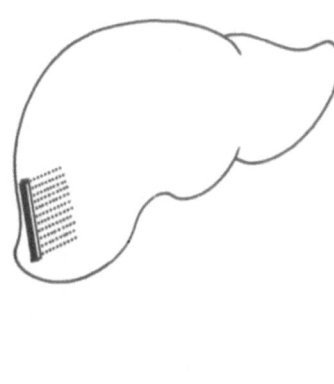

Figure 4.19. Liver Metastates.
A) A hypoechoic lesion (white arrow) along with a 'bull's eye' lesion (black arrow) are evidenced near the surface.
B) 1 cm (m) metastasis of endocrine tumor (carcinoid of the ileum). Intraoperative ultrasound pointed up, besides two larger palpable nodules, 3 other hidden lesions. Surgical resection was performed.
C) Metastasis (m) returning low-level echoes with areas of irregular echogenicity. The margin of a serous cyst is visible in the upper pole of the right kidney.

The polymorphic appearance of metastases at ultrasound and the fact that certain features mimic primary liver tumors often make differential diagnosis problematic. However experience has shown that certain ultrasound characteristics are helpful in indicating the presence of one type of neoplasm rather than another. The small, uniformly hyperechoic lesions, be they single or multiple, found on occasion close to vessels are invariably angiomas. Hyperechoic metastases are never uniformly echogenic and their contours are less well defined and regular than primary tumors. Small hypoechoic lesions are almost always metastases or small liver carcinomas, especially in cirrhotic livers. A thin hypoechoic halo surrounding the lesion is a characteristic feature of a small liver carcinoma; in the case of metastases the hypoechoic halo is thicker and more irregular, the confines between it and the surrounding tissue being difficult to distinguish – a finding that contributes to the hypothesis that this hypoechoic rim reflects the tissue atrophy induced by rapid tumor growth [43].

When lesions that pose queries for differential diagnosis are found during intraoperative investigation, an echo-guided biopsy can be performed using a special cutting needle (Surecut or Trucut) and the specimen sent for definitive histological examination.

Diagnosing intrahepatic lesions

Intrahepatic lesions of less than 1.5 centimeters are often not detected by conventional diagnostic methods including ultrasound, CT scan, and angiography [9, 23, 57], and may also not be discovered at surgical exploration of the liver, especially if the lesion is deeply ensconced in a cirrhotic liver whose parenchyma is known to be considerably harder than that of cancerous livers [42, 44, 45].

The higher frequency of intraoperative ultrasound probes affords greater resolution, thereby enabling visualization of lesions as small as 4–5 millimeters. This is especially true of hyperechoic lesions (Fig. 4.20).

A prospective study [19] was conducted in our department on 54 patients undergoing surgery for primary liver tumors (32 cases) or metastases (22 cases); 28 of these were cirrhotics. Most cases [48] were asymptomatic and initial diagnosis was made on the basis of ultrasound follow-up. Only 3 patients presented with clinical signs such as pain or palpable mass. In 3 cases an increase in CEA or alpha-fetoprotein did help to direct investigation. All patients underwent angiography (digital angiography in 35 cases), contrast medium CT scan as well as ultrasound examination of the liver – by the same team of operators – using a 3.5 MHz probe.

These findings were compared with the results of intraoperative ultrasound, surgical exploration of the liver and the histological findings on the operative specimen. Hepatic resection (18 segmentectomies, 11 left or right hepatectomies, 6 left lobectomies and 2 extensive hepatectomies) was carried

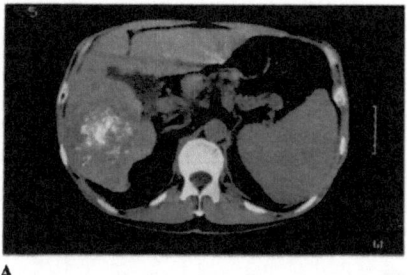

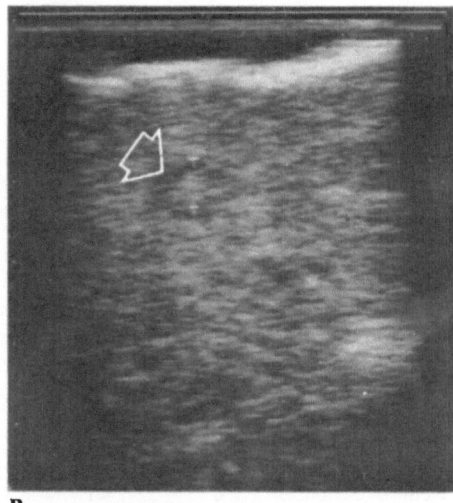

Figure 4.20. Small lesion not detected at preoperative examination.
Hepatocellular carcinoma on cirrhosis in the right liver lobe; neither preoperative ultrasound nor CT scan (lipiodol contrast medium) (A) showes other intrahepatic lesions.
(B) Intraoperative ultrasonography showes a small (6 mm) secondary lesion in the left lobe (arrow). (The examination was carried out using a gel pad.)

out in 37 of the 54 patients, while it was contraindicated in 17 patients, 4 of whom received in-dwelling catheters for chemotherapy infusion into the intrahepatic artery.

Table 4.1 compares the findings of intraoperative ultrasound with pre-operative techniques in cirrhotic and non-cirrhotic patients. Intraoperative ultrasound proved of greater diagnostic value than the pre-operative methods, especially in the case of small lesions. In fact the 2 lesions in the cirrhotic and the 2 in the non-cirrhotic group that intraoperative scan failed to detect were both less than one centimeter and immediately beneath the capsule. The most rewarding results were in the cirrhotic group where a con-siderable percentage of the lesions found were not palpable at examination.

Table 4.11 shows the sensitivity of CT Scan, angiography and preoperative ultrasound compared to intraoperative ultrasound (sensitivity means the number of lesions detected compared to the total number of lesions). CT Scan detects less than half the lesions under 2 centimeters and often fails to pick up small lesions in cirrhotic livers if their density mimics that of the parenchyma. Angiography only rarely evidences minute intrahepatic lesions, and when it has done, the lesions were prevalently highly vascularized metas-tases of endocrine tumours. Furthermore conventional, non-digital angiog-raphy often fails to detect even large hypovascular metastases unless in the left lobe. Even in the case of preoperative ultrasound, the limit would seem to be lesions of less than 1 centimeter and those located in the so-called 'blind areas' recently reported by Gunven and Hasegawa in their exhaustive

Table 4.1. Diagnosis of liver neoplasms

A) *Non cirrhotic liver (26 pts)*

Ø	No of lesions	CT	ANGIO	Preop US	Intraop US	Non palpable lesions
< 1 cm	6	3	1	3	4	3
1–3 cm	11	6	4	8	11	2
> 3 cm	27	25	24	26	27	–
Total	44	34 (77.2%)	29 (65.9%)	37 (84.1%)	42 (95.4%)	5 (11.3%)

B) *Cirrhotic liver (28 pts)*

Ø	No of lesions	CT	ANGIO	Preop US	Intraop US	Non palpable lesions
< 1 cm	5	0	1	1	3	4
1–3 cm	19	8	11	14	19	11
> 3 cm	10	8	8	10	10	3
Total	34	16 (47.0%)	20 (58.8%)	25 (73.5%)	32 (91.1%)	18 (52.9%)

Table 4.2. Sensitivity of different diagnostic techniques in the diagnosis of liver neoplasms

	Ø Lesion	CT (%)	Angiography (%)	Preop US (%)	Intraop US (%)
Non cirrhotic Liver	< 1 cm	50.0	16.6	50.0	66.6
	1–3 cm	54.5	36.3	72.7	100
	> 3 cm	92.5	88.8	96.2	100
Cirrhotic Liver	< 1 cm	0.0	20.0	20.0	60.0
	1–3 cm	42.1	57.8	73.6	100
	> 3 cm	80.0	80.0	100	100
	Total	64.1	62.8	79.4	94.8

review [23]: i.e. posterior segment lesions which may be masked by the ribs or pleura and very superficial lesions.

Apart from this study of patients undergoing liver surgery for neoplasia, another study has been carried out on the ability of intraoperative ultrasound to detect occult synchronous liver metastases in patients with digestive tumors. 110 patients operated on for gastrointestinal or pancreatic tumors were prospectively investigated. All patients had preoperative ultrasound carried out by the same operator (L.B.) and careful palpation of the liver at surgery. Additional information was obtained with intraoperative sonography

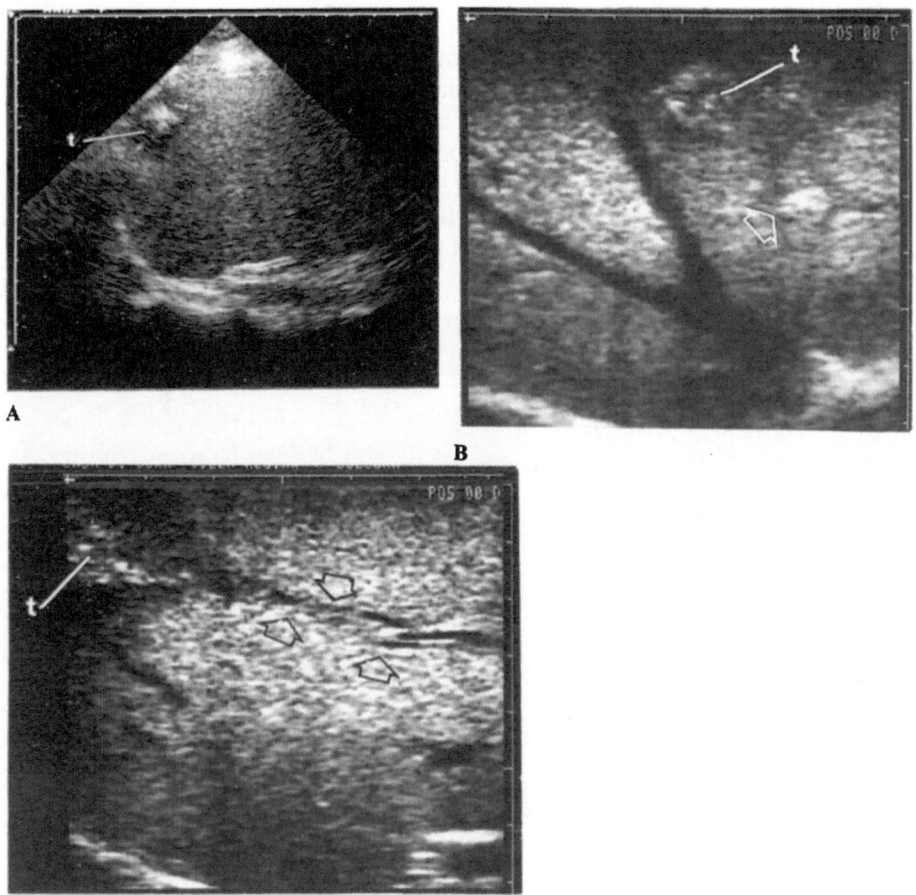

A

B

C

Figure 4.21. Intrahepatic lesions discovered in patient operated on for hepatic metastasis.
(A) Calcified hepatic metastasis in the 8th segment (t) detected at ultrasound control 2 years
after colectomy for cancer.
(B) Intraoperative ultrasound evidenced another smaller lesion (white arrow) and a neoplastic
thrombosis inside a portal branch (black arrow) (C).

in 8 patients. The sonograms of these occult lesions are presented in Fig.
4.22.

Two cases were typical target lesion images, of less than 1 cm and located
in the lateral segments of the right lobe of patients undergoing colon cancer
surgery. In both cases the metastases were removed with a wedge resection.
In 3 patients metastases were discovered at ultrasound during surgery for
pancreatic carcinoma. Concomitant dilatation of the intrahepatic bile ducts
may explain why these were missed at preoperative examination. One lesion
was an isoechoic mass on the posterior right lobe (Fig. 4.21). In the other two

cases the lesions were hypoechoic (Figs. 7.12, 7.13). In all cases the pancreatic resection planned as not carried out. Even large metastases may not be detected at preoperative ultrasound if situated in the posterior segments of the right lobe and hidden by the rib arch, especially in narrow-chested patients and where the liver is covered by the ribs and pleura. This was in fact the case in 2 patients with a metastasis of 3 and 4 cm respectively in the 7th segment. In these cases the tumor may also be difficult to palpate being covered by the insertion of the right triangular ligament (Figs. 4.22D, E).

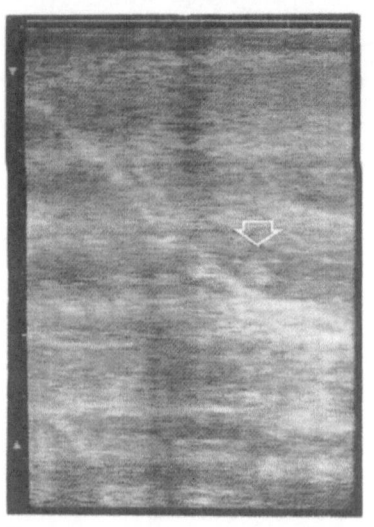

A

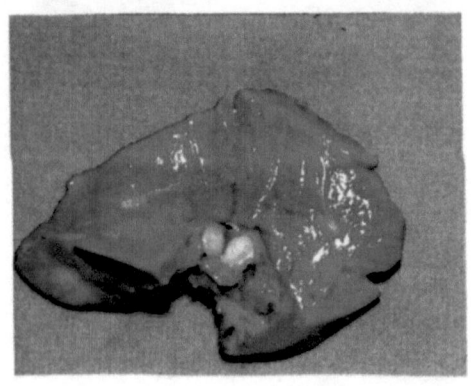

B

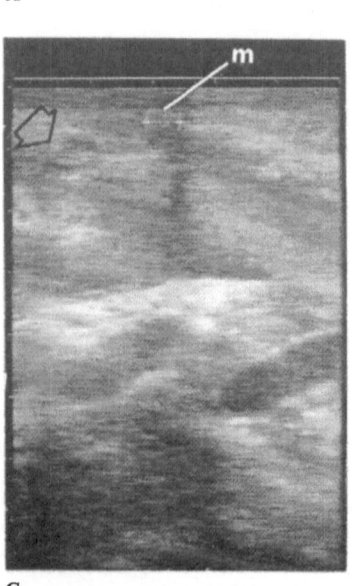

C

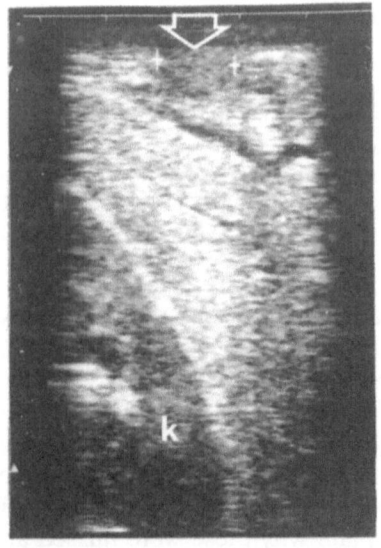

D

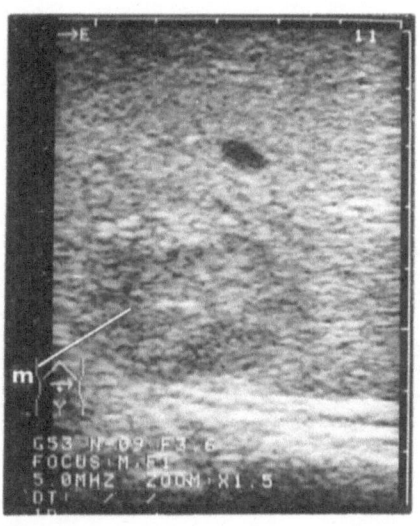 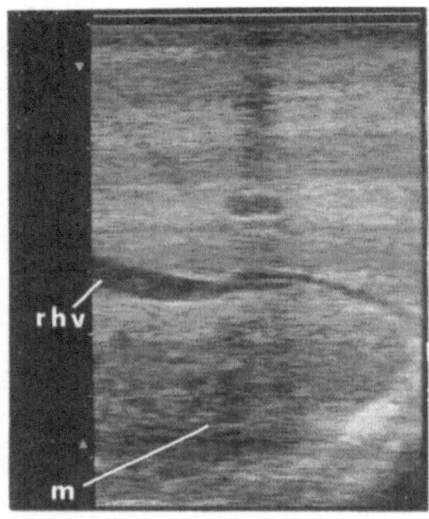

E   F

Figure 4.22. Occult hepatic metastases detected at intraoperative ultrasound in patient with
·digestive tumor.

A-B) Metastasis with 'target' lesion appearance (arrow) in the 6th segment in patient operated
on for colon carcinoma and removed with wedge resection.

C) Metastasis (m) of 5 mm of colon cancer visible in the left lobe of the liver. Note the neoplastic thrombus adjacent to the tumor in a segmental portal branch (arrow).

D) Isoechoic metastasis (1 cm) in a patient with pancreatic neoplasia, in the 7th segment
(arrow) above the upper pole of the right kidney (K).

E) Isoechoic metastasis (3 cm) in the posterior portion of the 7th segment at the point of entry
of the coronary ligament.

F) Large isoechoic metastasis (3 × 5 cm) in the 7th segment. Note the compression and shift of
the right hepatic vein. The tumor was palpable only after incision of the right triangular ligament.

Relationship of lesion to intrahepatic vessels

During surgery 3-D visualization affords good understanding of the extent to
which the lesion impinges upon or involves the intrahepatic, hepatic or portal
vessels. This can help avert accidental damage to major vessels during resection (Figs. 4.23, 4.24) as well as indicate when resection should be extended
to include vascular infiltration (Fig. 4.25) or where ablation is counterindicated if infiltration has gone too far (Fig. 4.26).

Not only can the lesion be accurately located in the hepatic segment but
also the afferent vessel can be detected along with the position of the adjacent
vascular peduncles. This enables exact anatomical excision of the segment to
remove all cancerous tissue while respecting the vessel branches of neighbor-
ing segments without needlessly sacrificing large tracts of hepatic parenchyma.

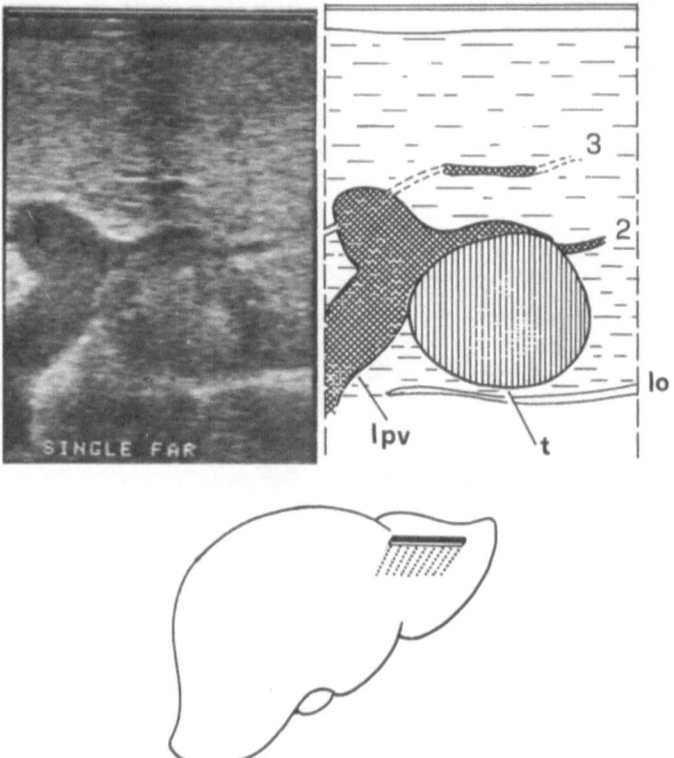

Figure 4.23. Small (2.5 cm) *hepatocellular liver carcinoma in a cirrhotic liver* in the 2nd segment adjacent to the left portal vein. A left hepatectomy was performed.

Consensus is growing over the need for segmental resection not only in the case of hepatocellular carcinomas on cirrhotic livers but also in liver metastases, since segmentectomies would seem to offer the same long term survival rates as major resections [5, 16, 17, 18]. Radical resection is being seen increasingly as recommended only for multiple lesions in one lobe or in the case of voluminous or central hepatic lesions [1, 33].

Figures 4.27 and 4.28 are examples of how intraoperative ultrasound can have a direct bearing on the surgeon's decision to perform segmental resection for liver metastases.

Another important feature of intraoperative ultrasound is its capacity to *detect neoplastic thrombi* in the main vessels or in the intrahepatic venous branches.

Neoplastic thrombi associated with liver neoplasms can be the result of either infiltration by a contiguous tumor, direct infiltration of the tumor into the endothelium of a vessel and subsequent break-away of centripetal thrombi [14] or – more frequently, especially in cirrhotic livers – the result of tumor invasion that will gradually work its way upstream from the segmental portal

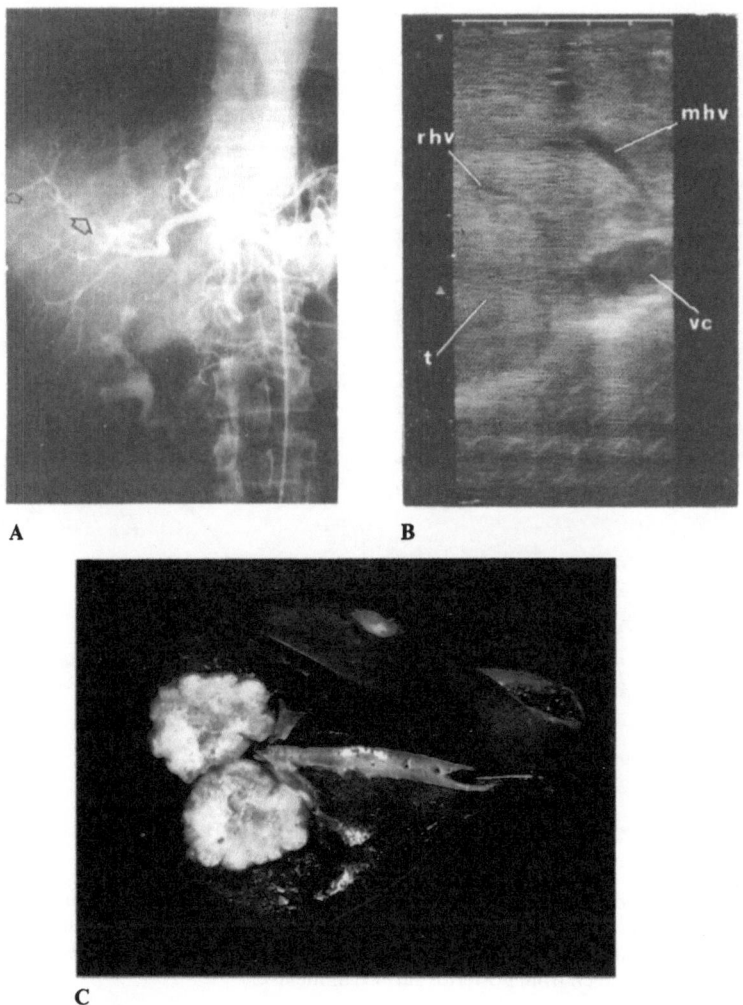

Figure 4.24. Large metastasis in segment 7.
A) Hepatic Angiography,
B) Despite tumor infiltration into the right hepatic vein near the point of entry more than 1 cm of normal parenchyma is clearly seen to separate tumor and vena cava. This made right hepatectomy feasible (C).

branch to the sectorial branch and then to the main trunk of the portal vein. This invasive pattern is enhanced by the spontaneous reversal of the portal circulation that sometimes occurs in liver cirrhosis and indeed, would account for the intrahepatic spread of an initially single-focus tumor [37, 41, 42].

This finding of intraportal neoplastic thrombi is very frequent in the literature from the Far East. Okuda [48] reports intrahepatic neoplastic thrombi in more than half the autopsies examined; Makuuchi [40, 42] found macroscop-

46

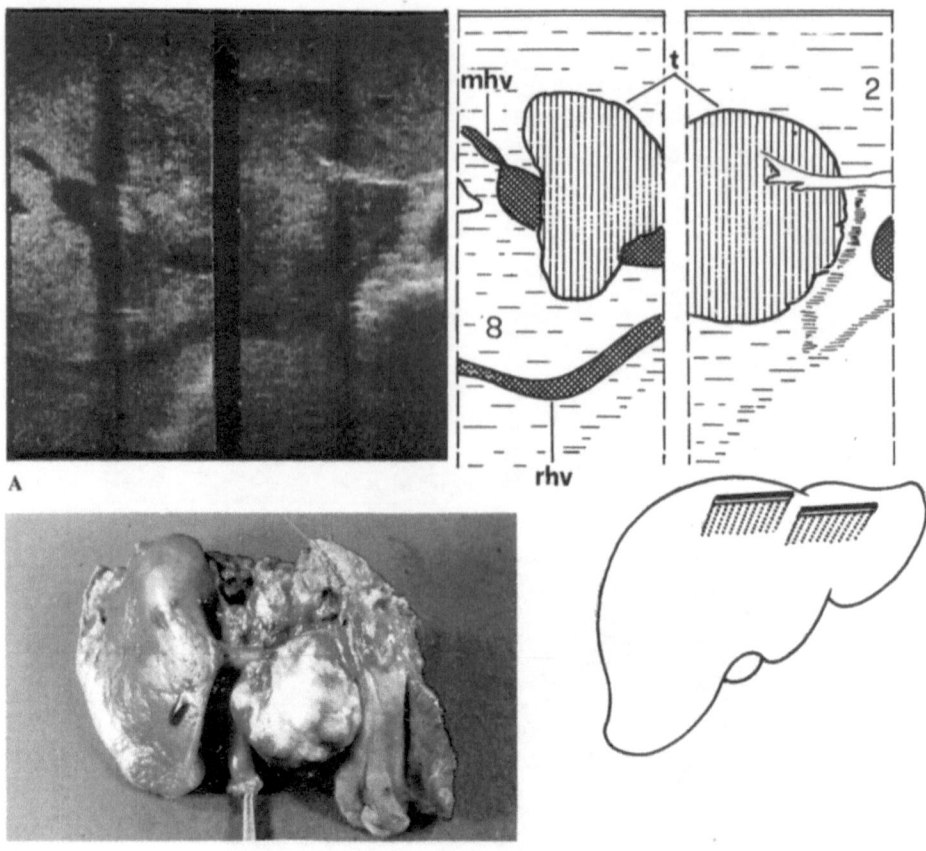

A

B

Figure 4.25. Large metastasis in the central portion of the liver mainly involving the caudate lobe and the 4th segment but also spilling over into the right of the middle hepatic vein towards the 8th segment (A). Ample left hepatectomy extended to segment 8 and 5 was performed.
B) Surgical specimen (seen from posterior surface of the liver).

ic thrombi in the intrahepatic portal branches in 15% of 62 cirrhotics undergoing liver resection for carcinoma. Moreover 3/4 of these patients were also found to have microscopic thrombi in the distal segment vessels. Similar data have been published by Yamazaki [66] and more recently by Igawa [27]. European and North American series [2, 15, 58], however, do not report such a high incidence of intraportal thrombi.

Of the 54 patients in our series, 4 proved to have intrahepatic portal branch thrombosis which was not, however, picked up at either arteriography or preoperative ultrasound examination. 3 were hepatocarcinomas in cirrhotic livers and one a metastasis of a colon primary.

In all cases, the caliber of the thrombosed portal branch was less than one centimeter. In three cases, the vessel involved was in a segment other than that

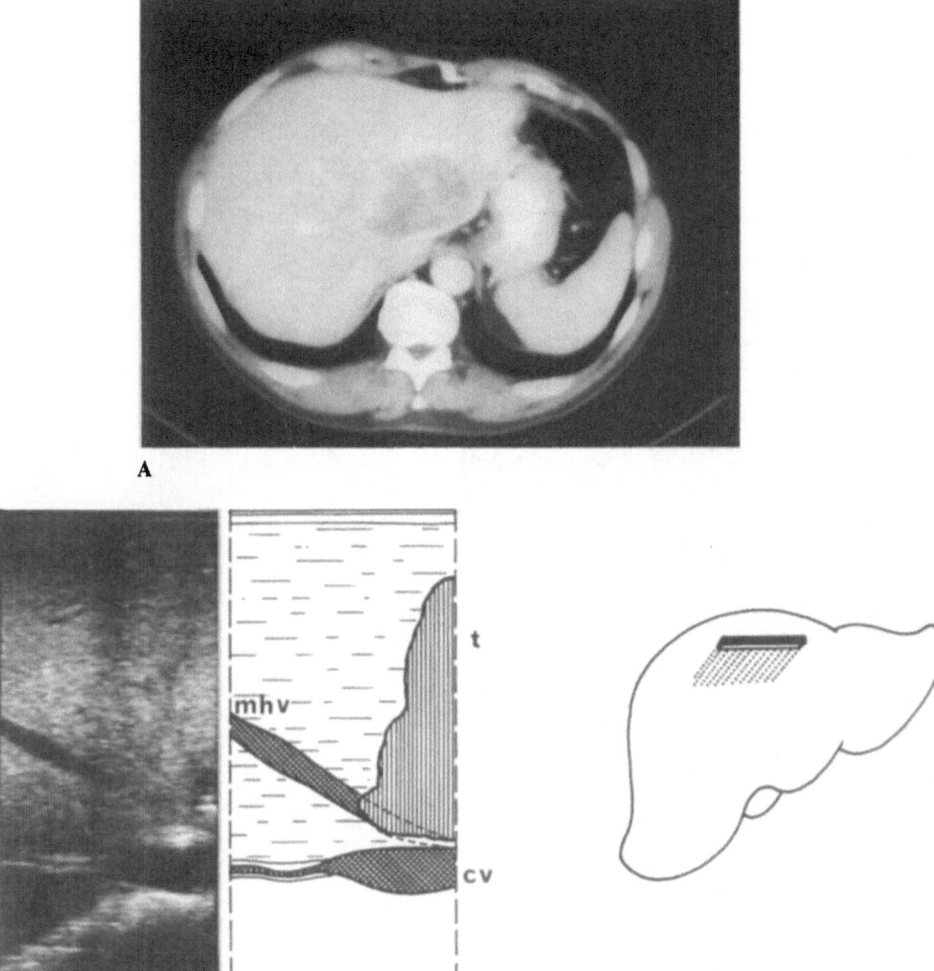

A

B

Figure 4.26. Recurrence of large liver metastasis. This patient had already undergone right hepatectomy to resect metastasis of colon cancer 16 months previously. Transabdominal ultrasound and CT scans (A) showed a focal lesion in the left lobe, while the liver parenchyma appeared completely regenerated, by and large resembling normal liver morphology.

B) Intraoperative ultrasound evidenced an area of irregular echoes with poorly defined contours extending from the point of entry of the sagittal hepatic vein into the vena cava. Note obliteration of the right hepatic vein. This US finding advised against the hepatic resection originally planned.

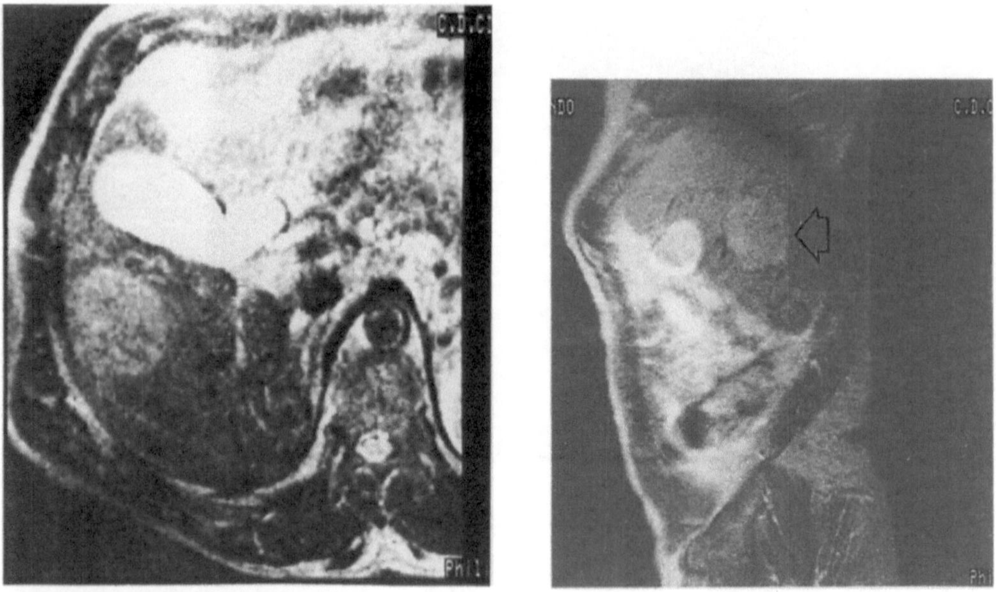

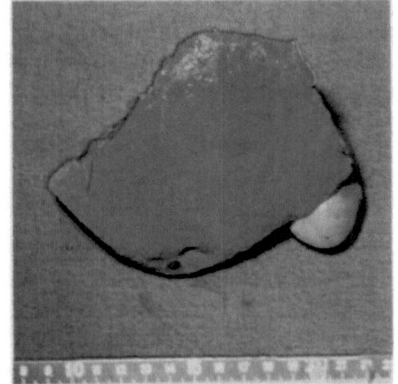

Figure 4.27. Hepatic metastasis of the left liver.
A, B) Nuclear Magnetic Resonance: transverse and sagittal scans. Lesion (arrow) located laterally and posteriorly to the gallbladder. Intraoperative ultrasound (C) allows exact location of the lesion in the 5th segment at some distance from the portal branches, thus indicating the feasibility of segment 5 resection.

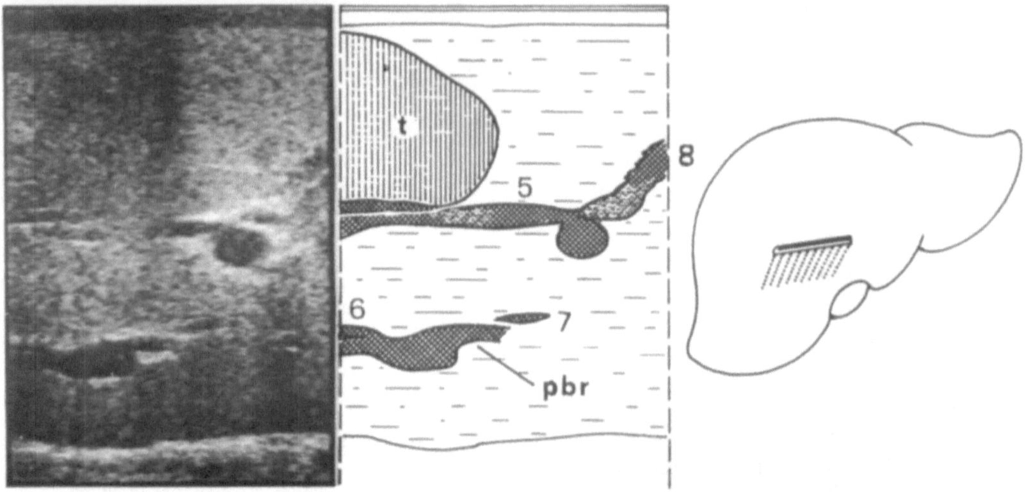

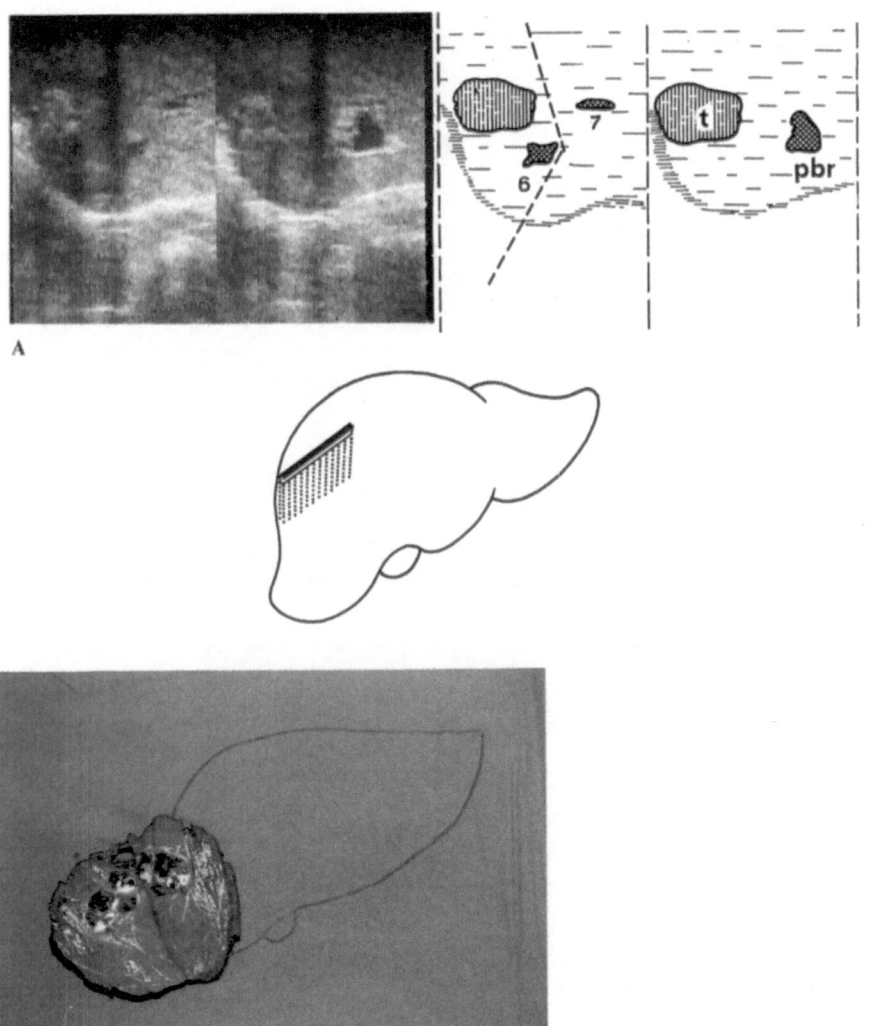

A

B

Figure 4.28. Liver metastasis of segment 6.
A) Intraoperative ultrasound shows the relationship between lesion (t) and the lateral portal peduncle (pbr); the branch of the 7th segment appears unimpaired and at some distance from the tumor.
B) Surgical specimen: segmentectomy of the 6th.

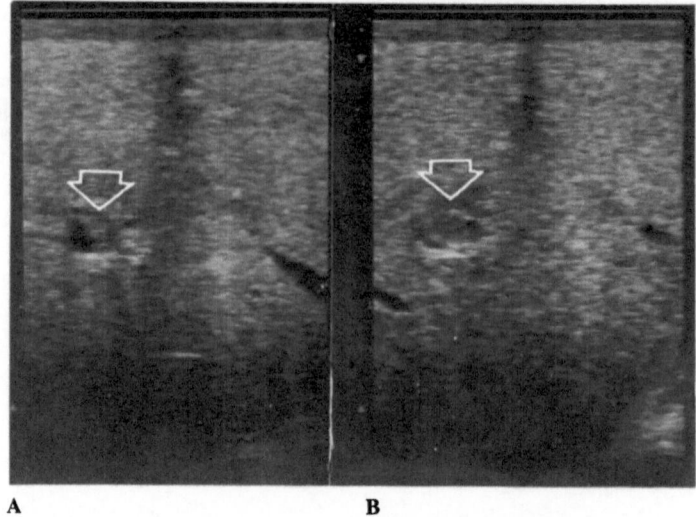

A   **B**

Figure 4.29. Neoplastic thrombosis (arrow) in a segmentary portal branch in a patient with hepatocellular carcinoma on cirrhosis. Partial (A) and total (B) occluding thrombosis.

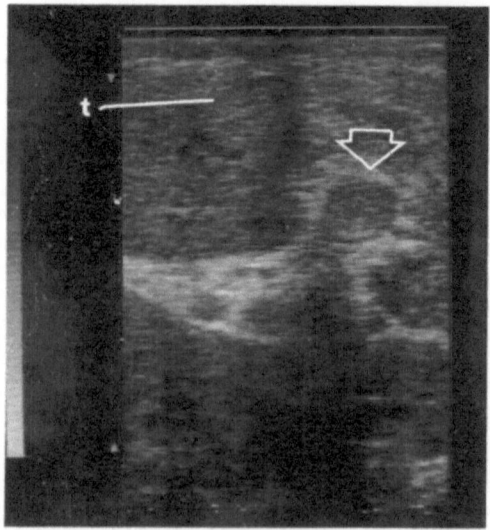

Figure 4.30. Neoplastic thrombus (arrow) in the terminal portion of the left branch of the portal vein. The tumor (t) can be seen in the 4th segment.

with the primary tumor (Fig. 4.29), while in 1 case the recess of Rex was thrombosed being adjacent to a tumor in the 4th segment (Fig. 4.30). In all 4 cases therefore, the hepatic resection originally planned was no longer feasible. Moreover, one patient – with hemorrhage from esophageal varices, taken to emergency surgery for porto-caval anastomosis – proved to have thrombosis of the inferior vena cava concomitant with liver carcinoma of the 6th segment (see fig. 9.2). This ultrasound finding prompted a change in surgical approach to stapler transection of the esophagus.

Surgery for liver carcinoma in cirrhotics

In recent years primary liver tumors have received increasing attention, not only due to a probable increase in their incidence [34], but more especially on account of the widespread availability of screening techniques such as ultrasound and the search for tumor markers in patients with chronic hepatitis or cirrhosis. In fact small hepatocarcinomas are being found with increasing frequency in cirrhotic livers [11, 21, 22, 54, 56]. The resultant increased demand for surgical resection in cirrhotics has meant that many, hitherto infrequent, surgical problems have become a routine occurrence.

The experience of Asian surgeons [24, 31, 35, 37, 46, 47, 50, 60] and the thrust given by people like Bismuth [5, 6] in Europe, have demonstrated that the risk of resecting cirrhotic livers is acceptable provided that reserve liver function is carefully assessed and removal of parenchyma be as conservative as possible [31, 36], which in turn presupposes accurate location of the tumor and appreciation of the involvement of intrahepatic vessels. This evaluation must of course be backed up by particular post-operative care [24].

This is where intraoperative ultrasound comes into its own, enabling the visualization of small tumors that escape detection at palpation or inspection of the cirrhotic liver. Nagasue [44] reports that approximately half the cancers of less than 4 cm actually present in cirrhotic livers cannot be palpated. Sheu [55] reports that intraoperative ultrasound was indispensable in more than 30% of cases, enabling limited resection of small unpalpable tumors in cirrhotic livers. In 9 of our cirrhotic patients, segmentary hepatic resection was possible thanks to intraoperative ultrasound scan which alone was able to locate impalpable tumor in the cirrhotic parenchyma (Table. 4.3).

Figure 4.31 illustrates some of these subsegmental resections of cirrhotic lesions to remove small tumors. Special techniques have been described for this type of echo-guided resection. For small tumors, the surrounding parenchyma and adjacent vessels are 'tatooed' [61] to enable subsequent recognition and ensure that resection includes approximately 2 cms of non-neoplastic tissue around the tumor (Fig. 4.32). Tobe [61], Hasegawa and Makuuchi [41] have introduced an interesting technique whereby methylene blue is injected into both the portal peduncle supplying the tumor and selected segments of the portal branch to visualize the whole district (Fig. 4.33). The

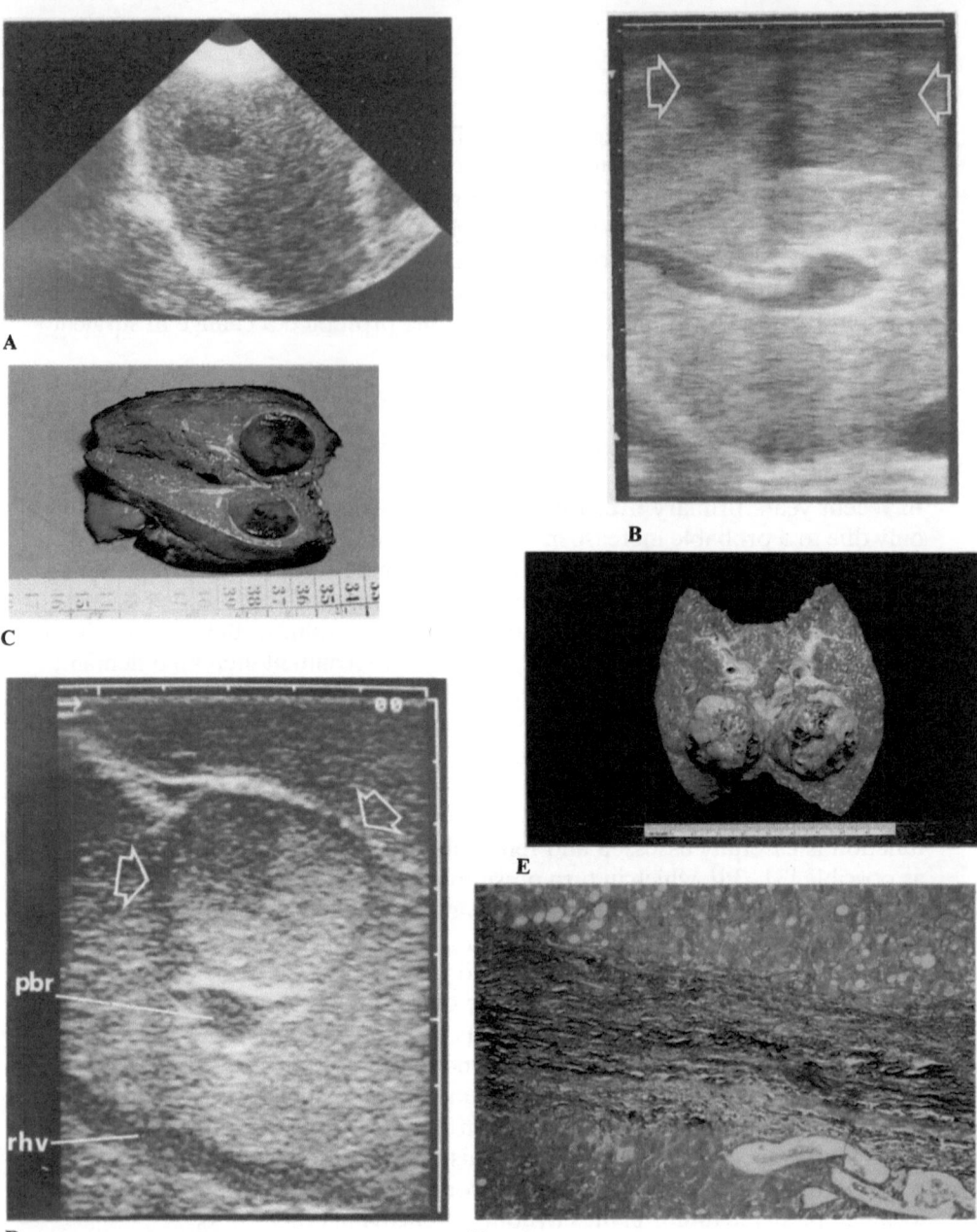

Figure 4.31. 'Echoguided' segmentectomies to remove small hepatocarcinomas in cirrhotic livers (Case no. 1).

A) Here routine ultrasound scan had evidenced a suspect nodule in the 6th segment, accompanied by a slight rise in alpha-fetoprotein levels (150 mg/100 ml).

B) Although not palpable at surgery, the nodule was evidenced at intraoperative ultrasound which clearly showed the presence of a hypoechoic peripheral halo (arrows).

C) Surgical specimen.

D) Hepatocellular carcinoma (diameter 3 cm) in Riedel's lobe contiguous to the portal bifurcation. The lesion (arrow), surrounded by a hypoechoic halo, has not invaded the portal branch (pbr) the walls of which appear highly echogenic and regular. Note the irregular course of the right hepatic vein due to underlying cirrhosis.

E) Resected piece.

F) Histologic finding clearly showing the capsule (Mallory, x264).

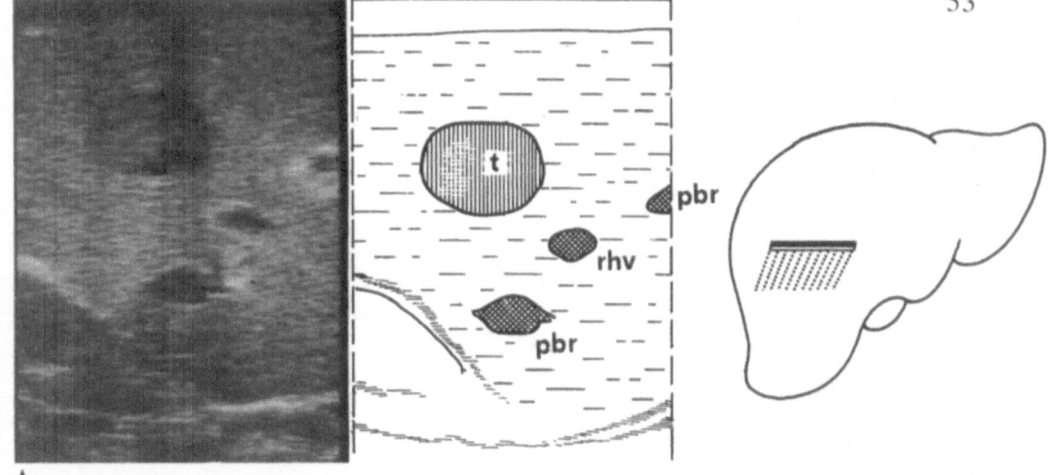

A

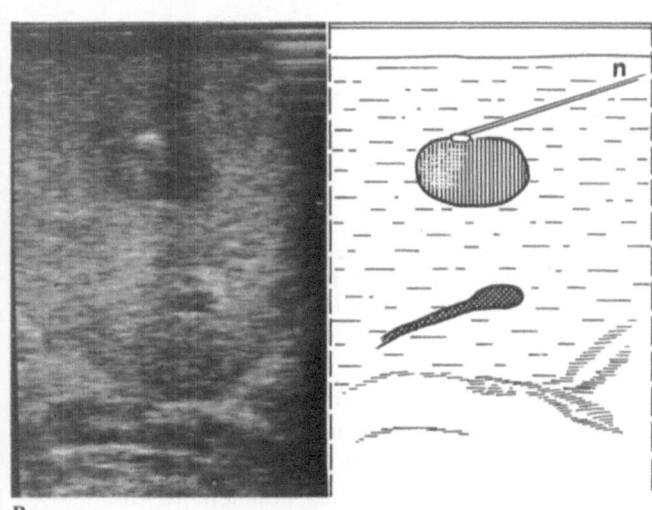

B

Figure 4.32. 2 cm diameter, non-palpable hepatocellular carcinoma in cirrhotic liver.

A) The tumor is located on the same scan plane as the right lateral scissure. Note the position of the right hepatic vein (rhv) and portal peduncles in the lateral and paramedian sectors (pbr). Right hepatectomy was not feasible as the patient was cirrhotic, nor was segmentectomy – given the position of the tumor.

B) To ensure removal of both tumor and a sufficient amount of peritumoral parenchyma, methylene blue was injected around the lesion to delineate the area for resection. Prior to surgery, the hepatic peduncle was clamped. The needle appears as a highly echogenic dotted image (B), while the stain returns strong reverberating echoes (C) on account of the gas bubbles in the liquid.

D) Surgical specimen.

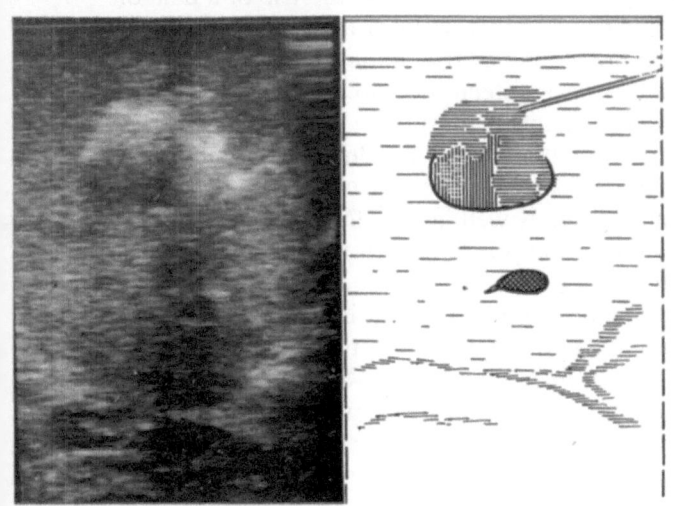

C

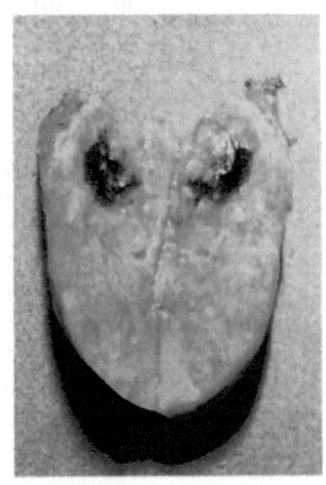

D

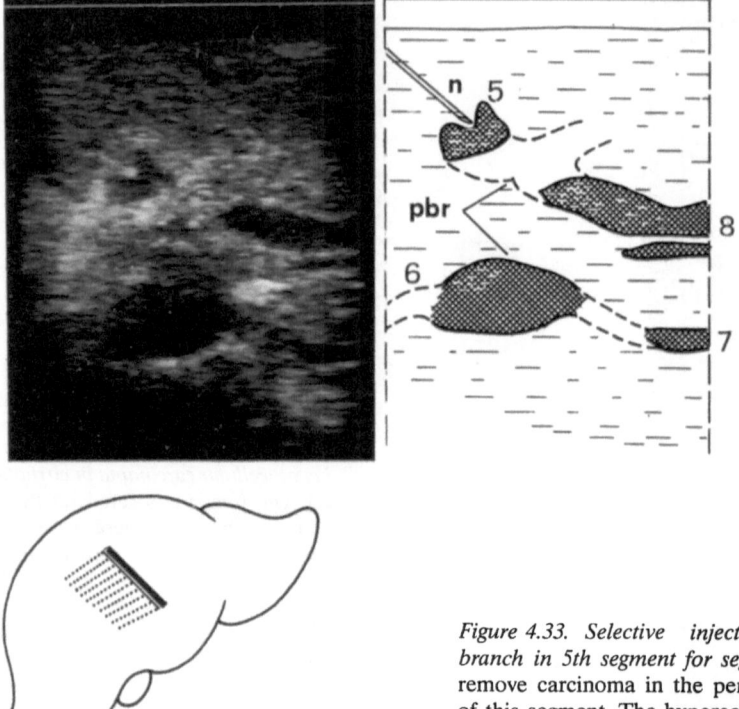

Figure 4.33. Selective injection of portal branch in 5th segment for segmentectomy to remove carcinoma in the peripheral portion of this segment. The hyperechoic needle can be seen clearly inside the portal branch.

rationale for this technique is the above-mentioned hypothesis that neoplastic emboli are transported up stream by the portal circulation, spreading first to that particular segment and then to the rest of the liver; it follows that hepatic resection must include all the segmental portal branches adjacent to the lesion [44]. Bismuth [8] has associated to this technique the use of a balloon catheter introduced into the segmental or sectorial portal branches and then inflated so as to interrupt blood flow to the district in question; if the hepatic artery is also clamped, bloodless segmentectomy can be performed with ischemia limited to the involved segment. It must, however, be said that we have never encountered severe difficulties when conducting resection with total clamping of the hepatic branch, and indeed Nagasue [46] reports that cirrhotic livers tolerate clamping perfectly well just as do non-cirrhotic livers [26]. Moreover, selective injection of the portal branch is not feasible in the case of tumors located centrally or along the central lobar fissure. ·

Another advantage of intraoperative ultrasound is that secondary tumor nodules can be evidenced even at some distance from the primary mass – a finding which would advise against hepatic resection. Satellite intrahepatic nodules (average diameter 1.3 cm), not seen at preoperative morphological examination nor palpated during surgery, were evidenced in 6 of our 28 cir-

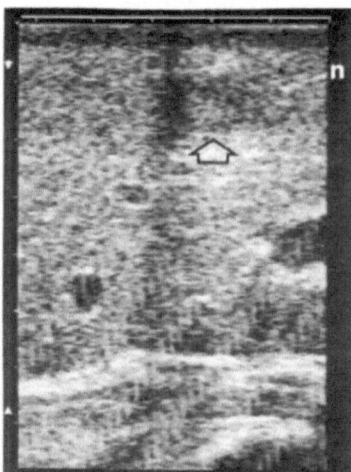

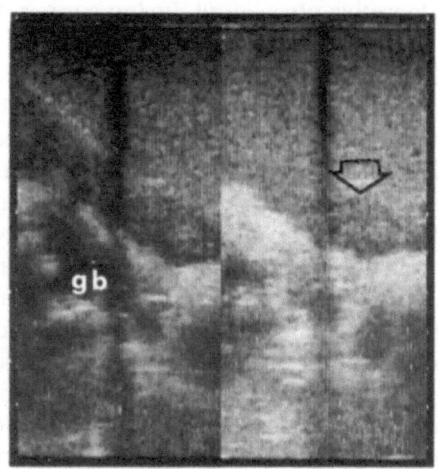

Figure 4.34. Small (1 cm) satellite nodule (4th segment – arrow) *of liver carcinoma.* The primary lesion was in the 7th segment. Biopsy was performed under u.s. guidance using a Surecut needle (n). The presence of a malignant nodule was confirmed, thus counterindicating resection.

Figure 4.35. Hyperplastic nodule in cirrhotic liver (arrow) but whose ultrasonic appearance was hypoechoic with ill defined contours and without a peripheral halo. Echoguided biopsy proved this to be a benign lesion.

rhotic patients, who as a result did not undergo hepatic resection (Figs. 4.14, 4.34; Table 4.3).

The advances in diagnostic techniques have brought another issue to the fore: *benign hyperplastic nodules in cirrhotic livers.* They appear as hypoechoic masses without a peripheral halo [51] and may easily be mistaken for a tumor [45]. Nor can they be recognised at palpation, having the same consistency as the cirrhotic parenchyma. Intraoperative ultrasonography permits ultrasound guided biopsy, and if the nodule proves benign, excision is counterindicated (Fig. 4.35).

Table 4.3. Influence of intraoperative ultrasonography on surgical strategy (54 cases)

	Primary liver tumors (32)	Metastases (22)
Hepatic resections (37)	9 Sub segmentary resections in cirrhotic livers	2 large hepatectomies
Contraindications to resections (17)	14 Multiple lesions: 6 Neoplastic thrombosis: 5 Benign lesions: 3	2 Multiple lesions: 1 Vascular infiltration: 1

Operative ultrasound during surgery for hepatic hydatidosis

Hydatid cysts have a characteristic ultrasonic appearance, presenting as rounded, predominantly anechoic masses with irregular areas indicating daughter cysts and echogenic septa and a well defined hyperechoic wall [9]. Diagnosis is readily carried out with transabdominal ultrasound, except in the rare cases of atypical cysts such as suppurated lesions which contain dense heterogeneous matter, or completely liquid filled cysts without septa or daughter cysts which may be mistaken for simple serous cysts, as in the case in Fig. 4.36. Here intraoperative ultrasound scan may be necessary to clinch the diagnosis, evidencing the presence of the typical proligerous pericystic membrane surrounding the liquid filled cavity.

In these cases operative ultrasound affords the major advantage of visualizing the cyst in relationship to the rest of the liver and showing to what extent the pericystic membrane impinges upon the main intrahepatic vessels. Such an overview is obviously essential for correct surgical approach.

Today there is increasing preference for more radical surgery in the management of hepatic hydatid cysts of the liver in order to lower the risk of recurrence and limit the often grave sequelae subsequent to mere emptying and drainage of the cavity [52]. Recently several authors have been instrumental in promoting techniques that remove the whole cyst and its membrane thus avoiding the problems that so often dog the residual cavity, such as superinfections, bile fistulae, possible exogenous vesciculation of the cuticola and failure of the cavity to reabsorb on account of the rigid skin-like membrane [4, 59].

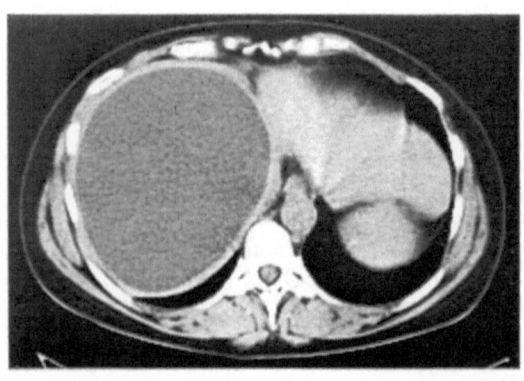
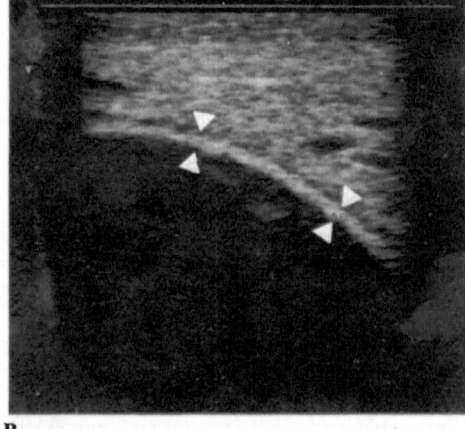

A   B

Figure 4.36. Hydatid cyst of the liver of completely liquid content.
A) CT Scan shows a large liquid formation with no septa or daughter cysts, occupying the whole right lobe of the liver.
B) Intraoperative ultrasound scan evidences a regular, highly echoic band clearly distinct from the surrounding liver parenchyma. This is the proligerous membrane. (Compare Fig. 3.2D).

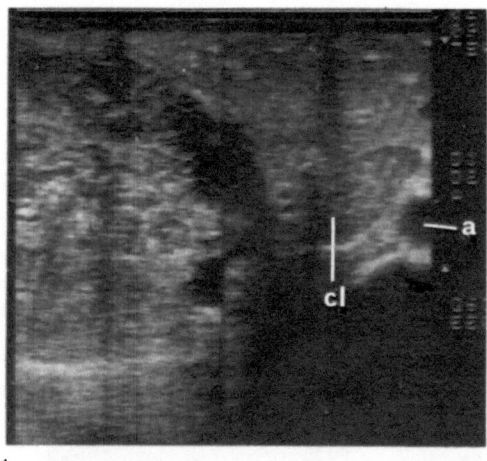 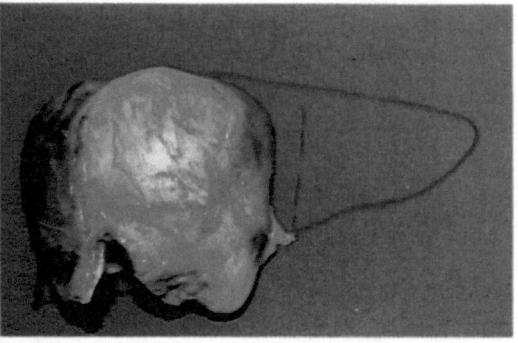

A **B**

Figure 4.37. Voluminous hydatid cysts containing several daughter cysts. The irregular echo-pattern mimics that of a solid mass. The left liver and caudate lobe (cl), behind which courses the vena cava, are disease free (A). The whole of the right lobe was occupied by the cyst and thus a right hepatectomy was performed. B) Surgical specimen. Compare with the appearance of a serous cyst (Compare Fig. 3.2D).

Intraoperative ultrasound is of special utility when deciding on the operative approach in hydatidosis since it shows the location of the pericystic membrane vis-à-vis the intrahepatic, hepatic and portal vessels as well as the vena cava lying behind the liver. The decision of whether to perform total pericystectomy, hepatic resection or simple drainage in the case of the cyst being dangerously near vascular structures, is taken on the basis of the findings in each specific case. Some examples of the role played by intraoperative ultrasound in guiding the surgeon in the management of hepatic hydatidosis are given in Figs. 4.37, 4.38, 4.39, 4.40, 4.41. This method is also all-important for the identification of bile fistulae and daughter cysts in the bile tract [8].

Liver abscesses

At ultrasound, liver abscesses present as largely hypoechoic formations with some irregular echoes. The contours are not easily distinguished from the surrounding parenchyma [9]. Although hepatic abscess is usually readily diagnosed with simple transabdominal scan, there are a few atypical forms, appearing ultrasonically as prevalently hyperechoic masses, that may be a problem to differentiate from tumor or suppurated hydatid cyst.

Today percutaneous drainage under ultrasound guidance is the treatment of choice for hepatic abscess [29, 30], while surgery remains indicated for chronic abscess with thick rigid walls but also for abscesses with dense, organized content and those in the dome of the liver on account of the difficulty

58

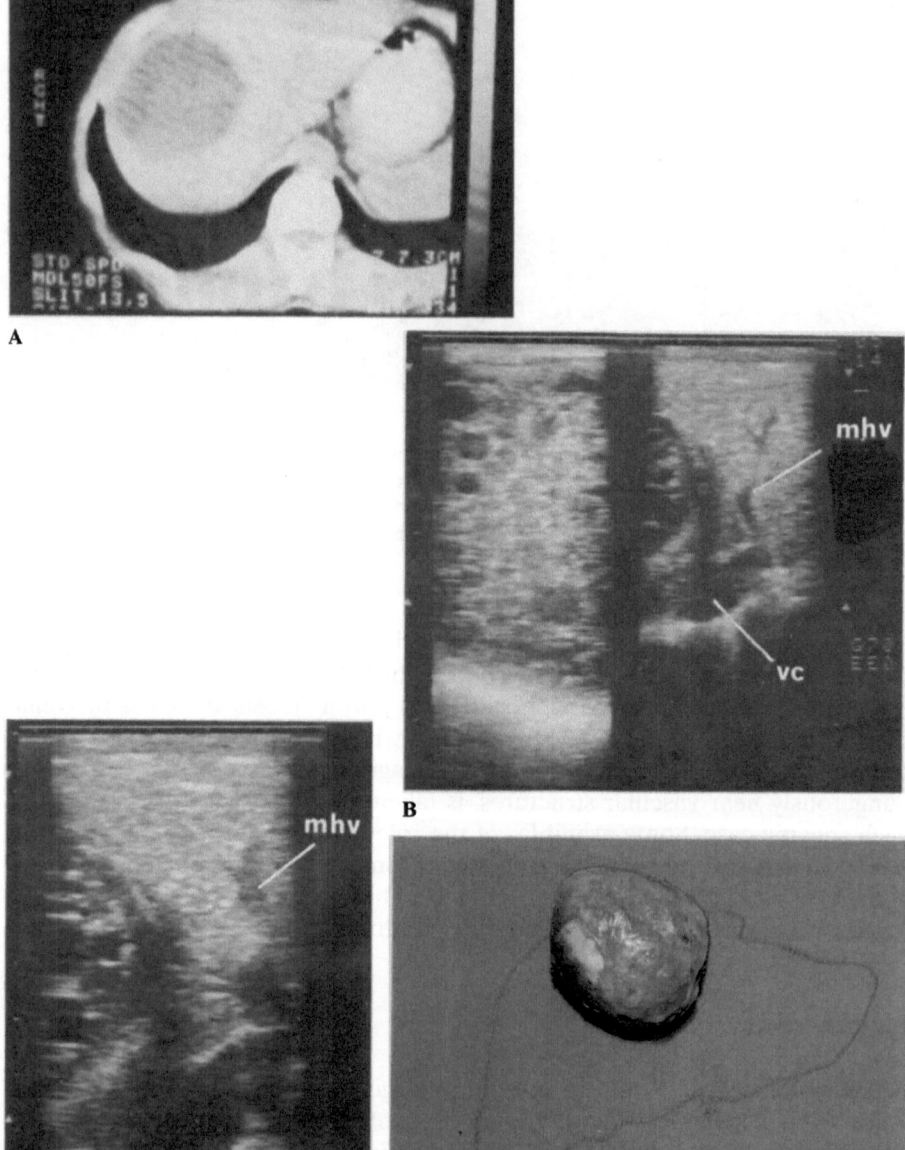

Figure 4.38. Hydatid cyst of the 8th segment.
A) CT Scan of the liver.
B) Adjacent to the vena cava and some 2 cm from the middle hepatic vein (C), this cyst presents a typical echo-pattern with rounded anechoic areas suggesting daughter cysts. Sub-total
cysto-pericystectomy was carried out (D), leaving a small portion of the pericystic membrane
near the vena cava in situ.

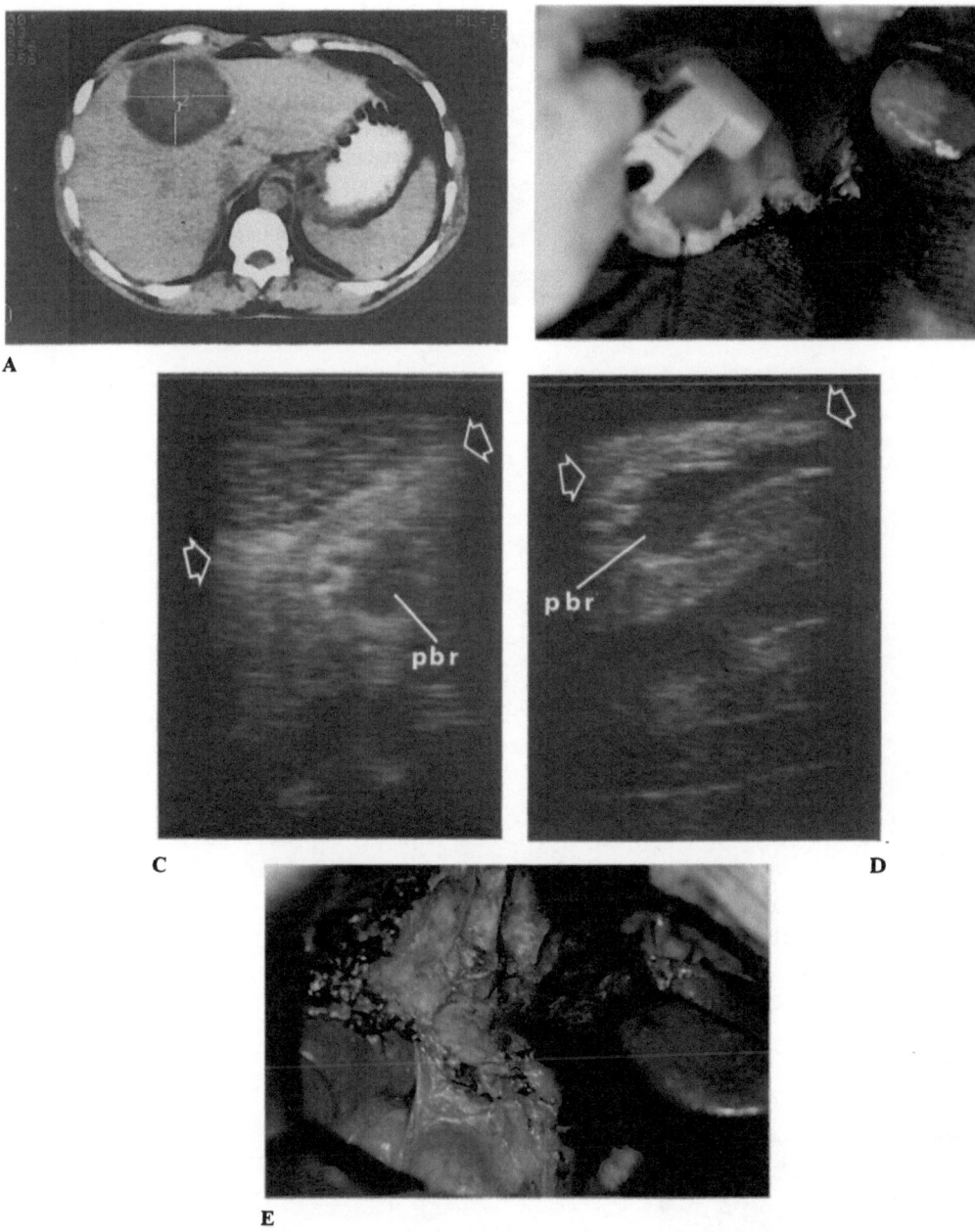

Figure 4.39.- Hydatid cyst of the 4th segment.

A) Liver CT Scan.

B) Intraoperative ultrasound after opening and draining the cyst. The cavity has been filled with saline solution and the probe explores the parenchyma from inside the cavity.

C, D) Several major portal branches (note the white triad consisting of the portal branch (pbr), the branch of the hepatic artery and bile duct) impinge upon the pericystic membrane (arrow). Partial pericystectomy was performed with cholecystectomy and resection of some 5th segment parenchyma to allow ample and uniform access to the cavity while the internal portion of the membrane contiguous with the intrahepatic vessels was left in situ (E).

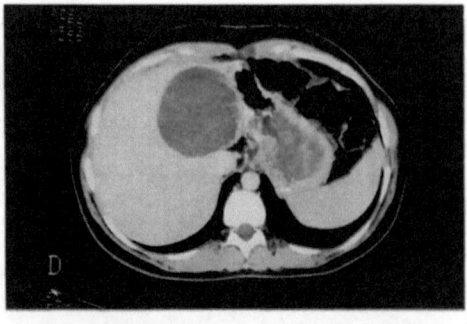

A

Figure 4.40. Hydatid cyst of the left lobe.
A) Liver Scan CT.
B) At intraoperative investigation the cyst is clearly seen to extend towards the right liver lobe and involve the right anterior portal branch (ant.p.br.) and especially the bile duct (bd). The cyst content is prevalently a solid mass comprising dead parassites.
C) Ultrasound control once cyst content has been removed and filled with saline. Note the close involvement of the anterior portal branch. The arrow indicates a bilary fistula which was sutured.

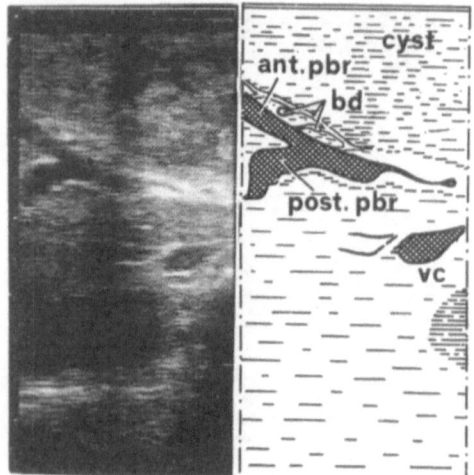

B

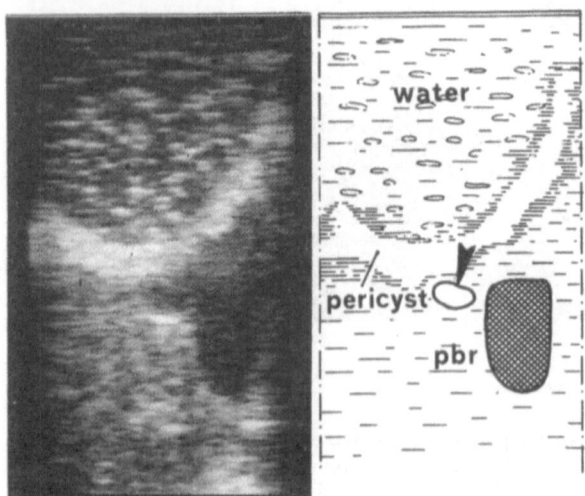

C

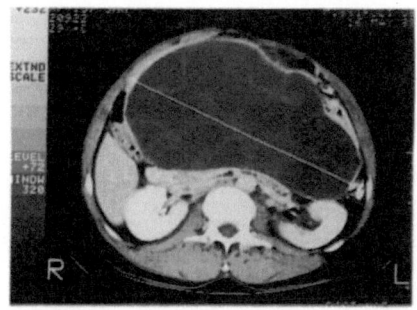

A

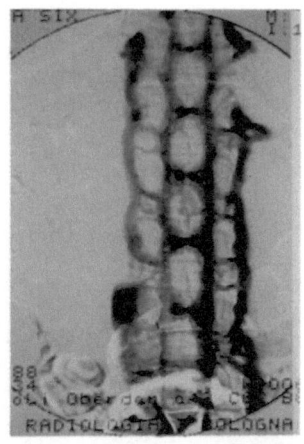

B

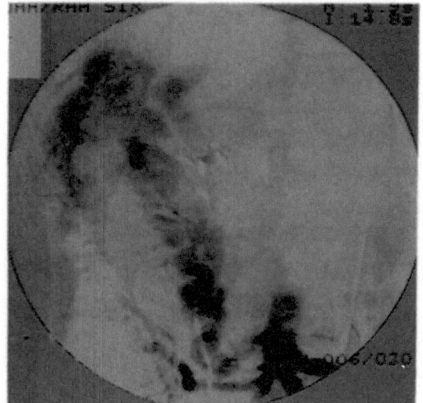

C

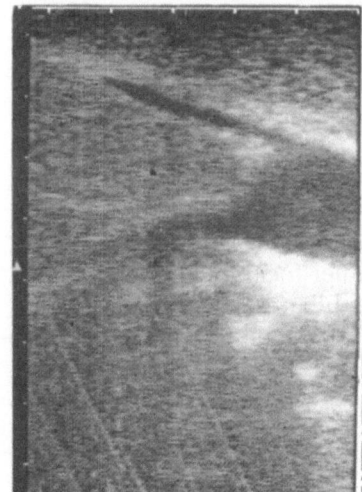

D

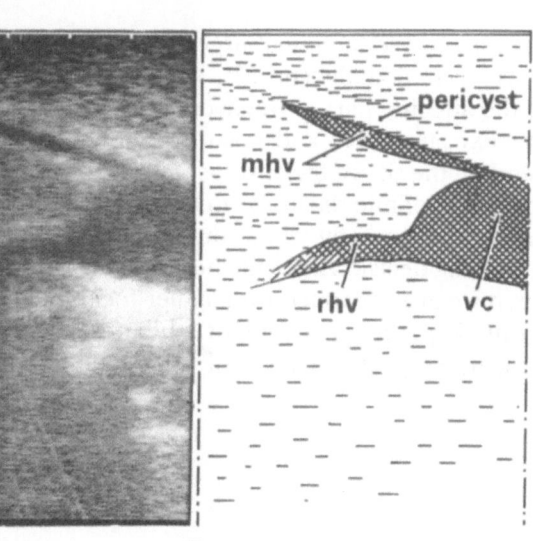

E

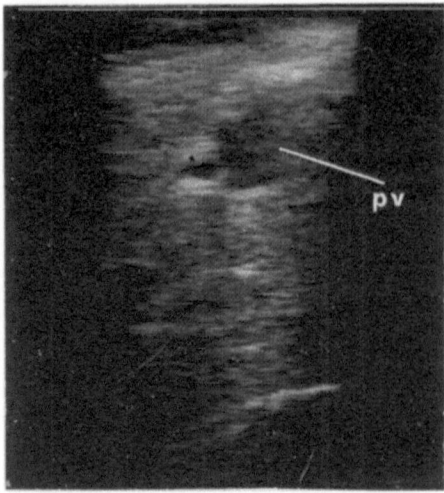

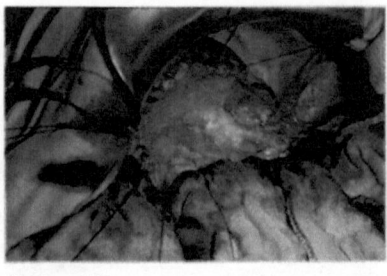

G

F

Figure 4.41. Huge hydatid cyst of the liver.
A) CT Liver Scan.
B) Cavography of the lower vena cava. Obvious signs of compression (or thrombosis) of the lower vena cava.
C) Arteriography of the mesenteric during venous return. The portal vein fails to opacify and there are numerous evident colalteral circuits.
D-E-F) After draining the cyst, the image from inside the cavity shows a patent vena cava and portal vein which are however in close connection with the peri-cystic area. This was removed under intraoperative echo guidance taking resection up to the limit of the intra-hepatic vessels (G).

in performing percutaneous puncture. Surgery consists of emptying and draining the abscess. Occasionally chronic, organized forms may require wedge resection of the affected part of the liver. However, since it is essential not to damage vascular structures and ensure optimum drainage, surgical technique will depend on the site of the abscess [52].

As well as establishing definite diagnosis in the atypical forms, intraoperative ultrasound can pinpoint exactly where the abscess is in relation to contiguous vessels, thus aiding decision as to the best drainage approach. The rest of the liver parenchyma can be scanned for smaller foci [38] and the draining and lavaging procedure kept under surveillance. Figures 4.42 and 4.43 are an example of 'echoguided' surgical drainage of a large abscess in the hepatic dome.

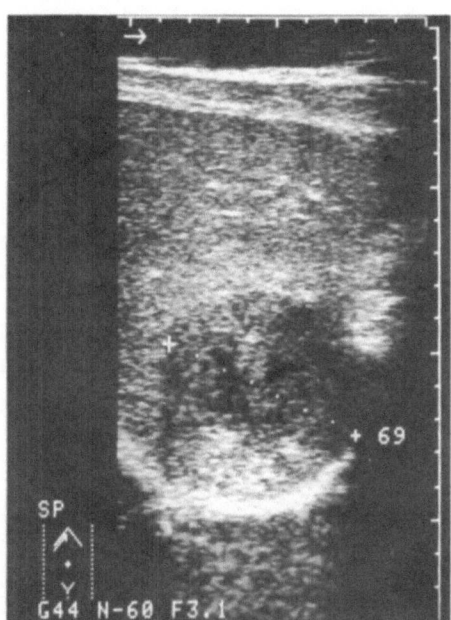

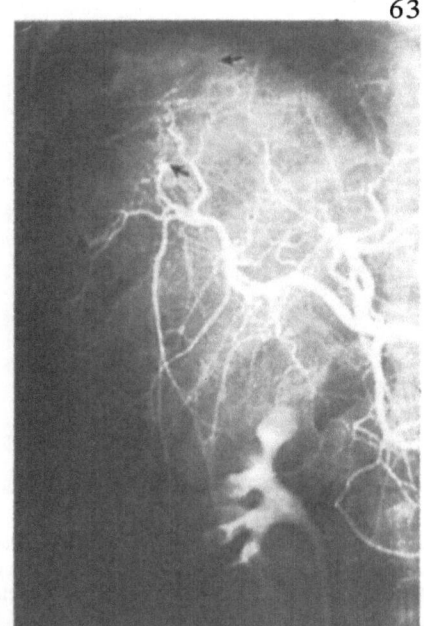

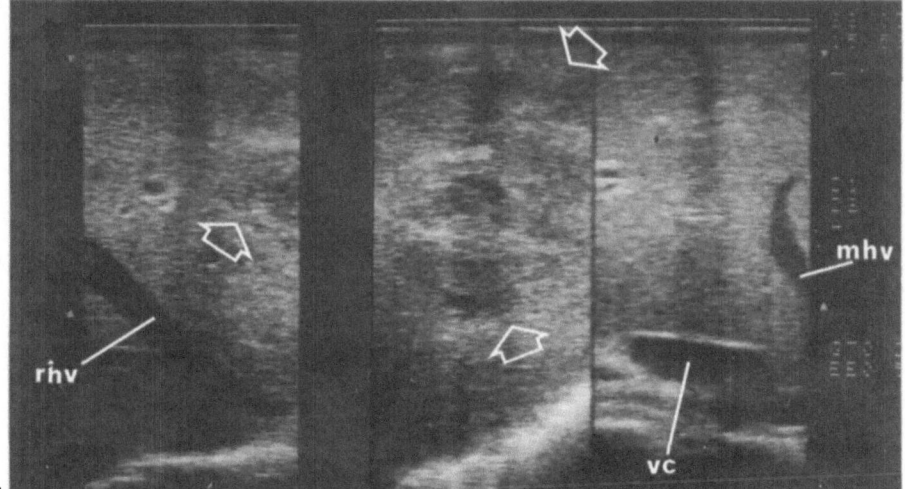

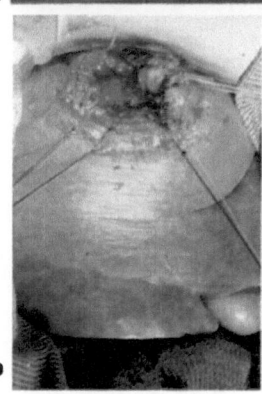

Figure 4.42. Liver abscess.
A) Transabdominal ultrasound scan shows a 6.9 cm lesion with a complex echo-pattern, located in the hepatic dome. As the ultrasound aspect was somewhat atypical, arteriography was performed which evidenced (arrow) an avascular area in the 8th segment (B).
C) intraoperative ultrasound confirms the presence of an area with anomalous echo-pattern with ill defined contours lying next to the right hepatic vein at some distance from the vena cava. Surgery consisted of abscess drainage with a wide aperture on the dome (D).

64

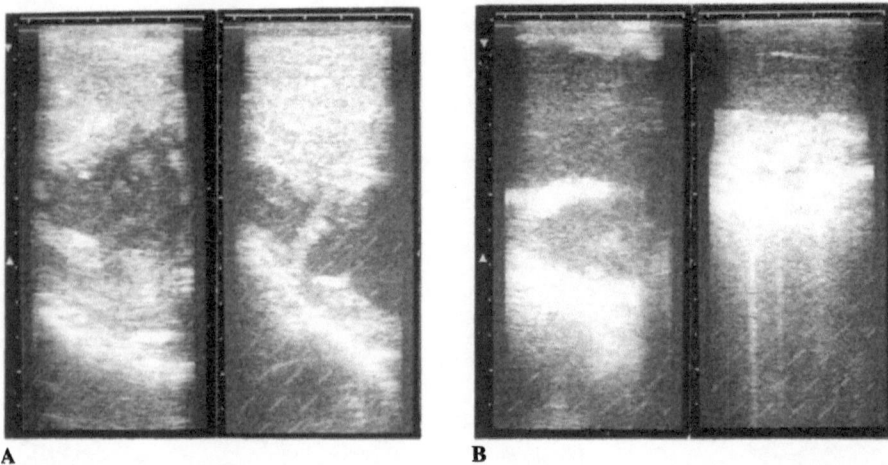

A   **B**

Figure 4.43. Recurrence of an amboebic abscess in a patient having already undergone unsuccessful percutaenous drainage of an abscess of inhomogeneous appearance (A) with septa (B). Ultrasound indicates where the abscess is closest to the surface of the liver, which will be the area for surgical incision.

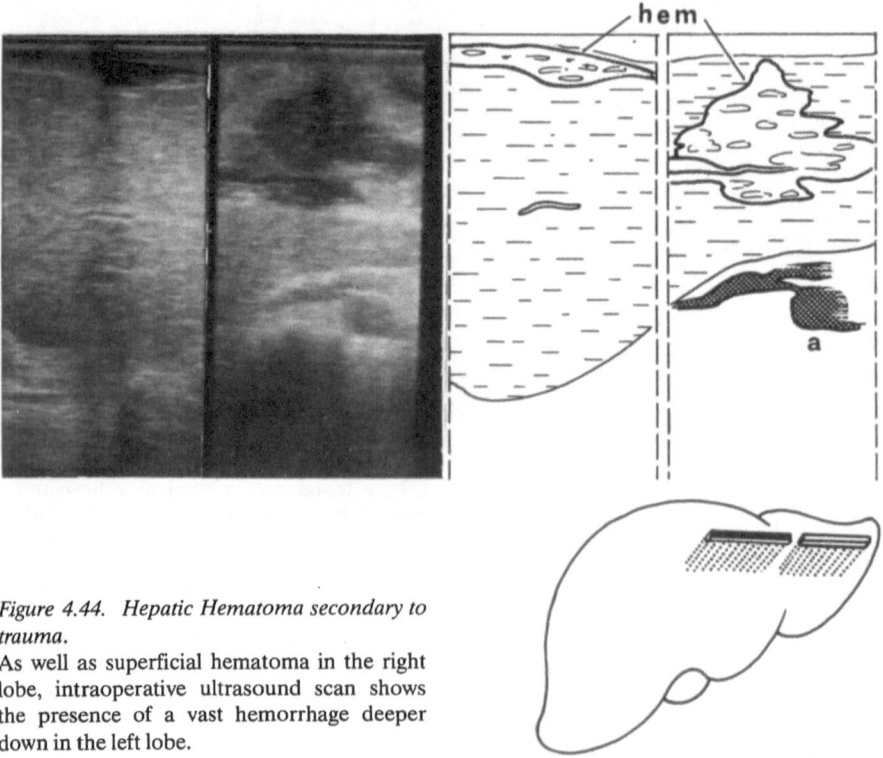

Figure 4.44. Hepatic Hematoma secondary to trauma.
As well as superficial hematoma in the right lobe, intraoperative ultrasound scan shows the presence of a vast hemorrhage deeper down in the left lobe.

Intraoperative ultrasound in traumatic liver lesions

Intraoperative scan of a traumatized liver allows the surgeon to take stock
swiftly and accurately of the extent of the damage. This is all the more important if there has been no time to X-ray the patient prior to preparation for
surgery. Superficial liver lesions may obscure deeper, central lesions that will
induce hemoperitoneum or embolism. Figure 4.44 shows an intraoperative
scan taken during emergency operation for hemoperitoneum secondary to
liver trauma. Surgical exploration evidenced a superficial lesion with lacera-
tion of the capsule and hematoma of the strata immediately underlying the
capsule; operative ultrasound scan, however, showed, hidden by the superficial hematoma, a vast centrally located hematoma extending through the
whole of the 4th segment right up to the left lobe and which was hemorrhag-
ing badly. The consequent decision in this case was to perform a left hepatectomy.

Even in the case of delayed surgery of traumatized livers, for example post
traumatic hemobilia, intraoperative ultrasound can be a most useful tool (see
Fig. 4.45).

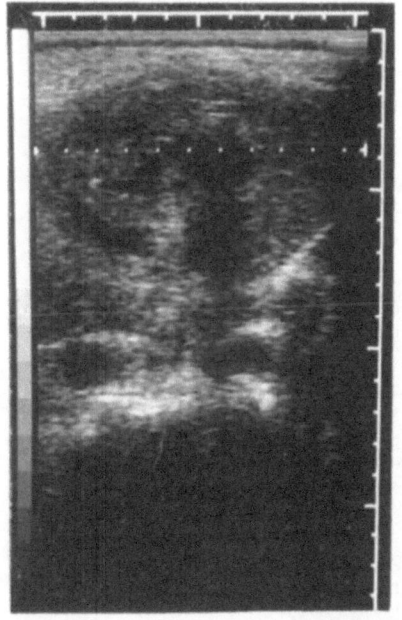

A

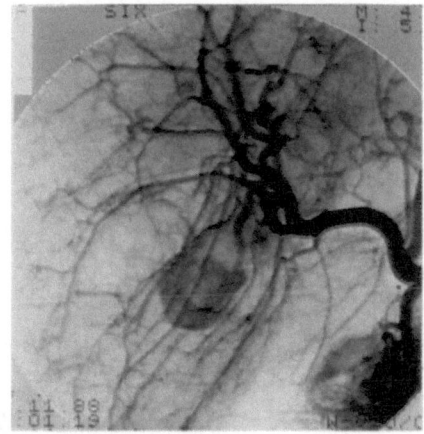

B

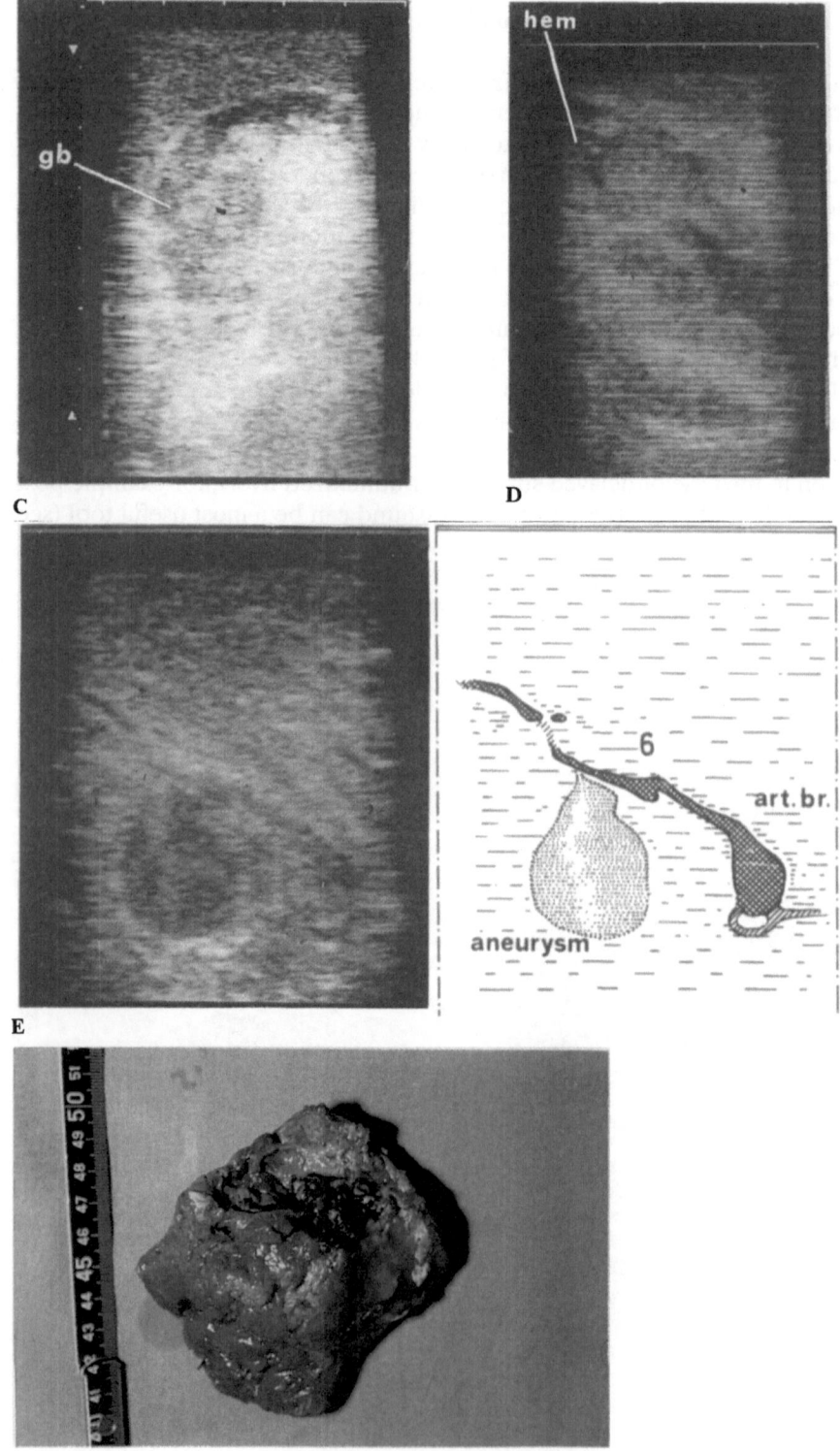

C

D

E

F

Surgical removal of benign liver tumors

Today benign tumors of the liver are seldom managed surgically. Apart from adenomas, which tend to grow spontaneously with risk of rupture, angiomas and focal nodular hyperplasia rarely tend to enlarge, the risk of rupture being

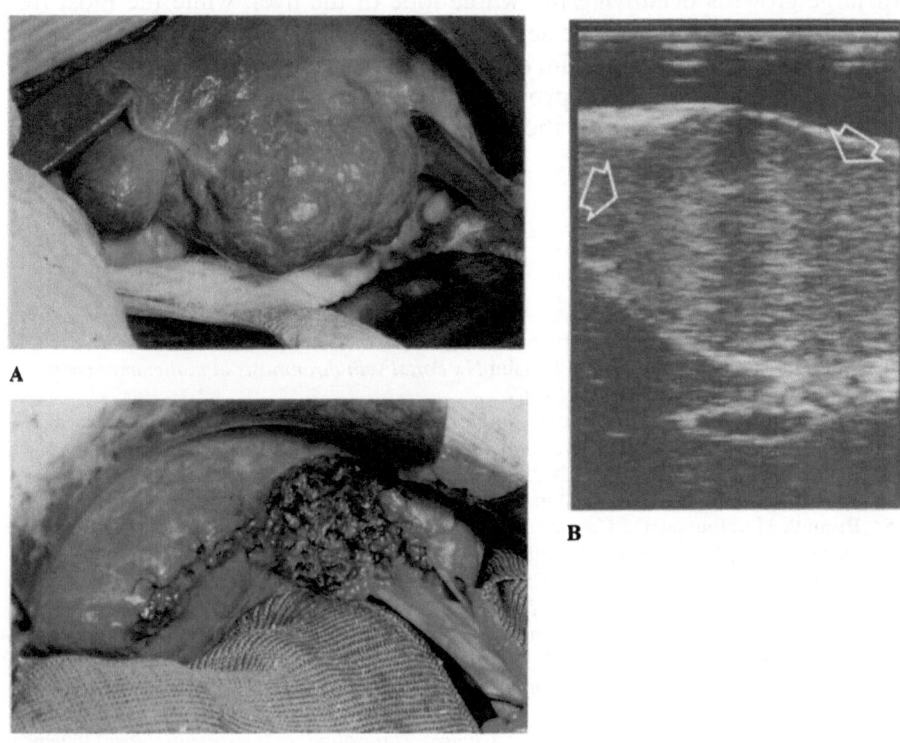

A

B

C

Figure 4.46. Angioma of the 4th segment.
A) Intraoperative picture.
B) Intraoperative scan using a gel pad. The angioma appears as a smoothly marginated, uniform, hyperchoic mass.
C) Operative field after resection of Riedel's lobe.

Figure 4.45. Post-traumatic Hemobilia.
22 year old patient, previously operated on for hemoperitoneum due to apparent sub-capsular rupture of the lateral segments of the right lobe of the liver. 20 days subsequently she presented digestive hemorrhage. Transabdominal ultrasound showed a vast inhomogeneous lesion in segment 6 which was a hepatic hematoma (A). Hepatic arteriography showed a post-trauma aneurism of an artery in segment 6 (B). Surgical exploration evidenced no palpable or visible lesions. Intraoperative ultrasound confirmed the diagnosis of hemobilia showing clots inside the gallbladder (C) as well as the vast inhomogeneous area of the hematoma in segment 6 (D). Also clearly visible is the aneurism originating in the arterial branch of the 6th segment and the turbulent blood flow set up (E). Segmentectomy of segment 6 was carried out including the aneurism under echo guidance to assess the correct plane of resection.

68

indeed very slight and decidedly overestimated in the past [25, 64]. They are hence only candidates for surgery if really symptomatic and obviously growing [20, 28].

In the case of surgery being performed, however, the benign nature of the tumor must be borne in mind. Thus major hepatectomies are only indicated for large growths occupying the whole lobe of the liver, while the most frequent type of exeresis will be segmental or an atypical section to excise just the tumor itself with a minimum of surrounding tissue [28].

Again intraoperative scan proves highly useful during segmental surgery to delineate the exact extent of the intrahepatic tumor and the involvement of vessels (Fig. 4.46).

References

1. Adson M. A., Van Heerden J. A., Adson M. H. et al.: *Resection of hepatic metastases from colorectal cancer.* Arch. Surg. 119: 647–651, 1984.
2. Albacete R. A., Matthewes M. J., Saini N.: *Portal vein thrombosis in malignant hepatoma.* Ann. Intern. Med. 67: 337–342, 1967.
3. Belghiti J., Cardi F., Men Y. et al.: *Surgical treatment of hepatocellular carcinoma in cirrhosis. Value of peroperative ultrasonography.* Gastroenterol Clin. Biol. 10: 224–247, 1986.
4. Belli L., Del Favero E., Marni A., Romani F.: *Resection versus pericystectomy in the treatment of hydatidosis of the liver.* Am. J. Surg. 145: 239–242, 1983.
5. Bismuth H., Houssin D., Castang D.: *Major and minor segmentectomies 'réglées' in liver surgery.* World J. Surg. 6: 10–17, 1982.
6. Bismuth A., Houssin D., Michel F.: *Le risque opératoire des hépatectomies. Expérience sur 154 hépatectomies.* Chirurgie 109: 342–348, 1983.
7. Bismuth H., Castaing D., Kunstlinger: *Ecographie peropératoire du foie et des voies biliaires.* Presse Méd. 13: 1819–1822, 1984.
8. Bismuth H., Castaing D.: *Echographie peropératoire du foie et des voies biliaires.* Flammarion Médicine-Sciences, Paris, 1985.
9. Bolondi L., Gandolfi L., Labò G.: *Clinical Ultrasound in Gastroenterology.* Piccin – Butterworths, Padova, 1984.
10. Castaing D., Edmong J., Kustlinger F., Bismuth H.: Utility of operative ultrasound in the surgical management of liver tumors. Ann. Surg. 204: 600–605, 1986.
11. Cottone M., Marceno M. P., Marigini A. et al.: *Ultrasound in the diagnosis of hepatocellular carcinoma associated with cirrhosis.* Radiology 147: 517–519, 1983.
12. Couinaud C.: *Le foie: études anatomiques et chirurgicales.* Masson, Paris, 1957.
13. Couinaud C.: *Controlled hepatectomies and exposure of the intrahepatic bile ducts. Anatomical and technical study.* C. Couinaud Ed, Paris, 1981.
14. Ebara M., Ohto M., Shinagawa T., Sugiura N., Okuda K. et al.: *Natural history of minute hepatocellular carcinoma smaller than three centimeters complicating cirrhosis.* Gastroenterology 90: 289–98, 1986.
15. Edmondson H. A., Steiner P. E.: *Primary carcinoma of the liver a study of 100 cases among 48900 autopsies.* Cancer 7: 462, 1954.
16. Fortner J. G., Silva J. S., Golbey R. B. et al.: *Multivariate analysis of a personal series of 247 consecutive patients with liver metastases from colorectal cancer. I: treatment by hepatic resection.* Ann. Surg. 199: 306–31, 1984.
17. Foster J. H.: *Survival after liver resection for secondary tumors.* Am. J. Surg. 135: 389–394, 1978.

18. Gennari L., Doci R., Bozzetti F., Bignami P.: *Surgical treatment of hepatic metastases from colorectal cancer.* Ann. Surg. 203: 49–54, 1986.

19. Gozzetti G., Mazziotti A., Bolondi L., Cavallari A., Casanova P., Grigioni W., Bellusci R., Villanacci V., Labò G.: *Intraoperative ultrasonography in surgery for liver tumors.* Surgery 99: 573–529, 1986.

20. Gozzetti G.: *Gli angiomi del fegato.* Atti Soc. It. Chir., Masson Italia Ed. Milano, Vol. I, 1986.

21. Gozzetti G., Mazziotti A., Cavallari A., Bellusci R.: *La chirurgia degli epatocarcinomi su cirrosi.* Massòn It. Ed., Milano, 1987.

22. Gozzetti G., Mazziotti A., Cavallari A., Bellusci R., Bolondi L., Grigioni W., Bragaglia R., Grazi G. L.: *Clinical experience with liver resections for hepatocellular carcinoma in patients with cirrhosis.* Surg. Gynecol. Obstetr. 166: 503–510, 1988.

23. Gunven P., Makuuchi M., Takayash K., Moriyama N., Yamasaki S., Hasegawa H.: *Preoperative imaging of liver metastases, comparison of angiography, CT scan and ultrasonography.* Ann. Surg. 202: 573–579, 1985.

24. Hasegawa H., Yamazaki S., Makuuchi M., Shimamura Y.: *The surgery of hepatocellular carcinoma associated with cirrhosis, with special reference to surgical techniques and pre, peri, post-operative care.* In: 'I tumori del fegato' G. Gozzetti et al., Editrice Compositori, Bologna, pp. 155–166, 1985.

25. Huguet C., Moujel J.: *Tumeurs primitives du foie chez l'adulte.* Masson Ed., Paris, 1983.

26. Huguet C., Delva E., Parc R., Hannoun, Camus Y., Bahnini A., Nordlinger B.: *Experience with 153 liver resections during the last 6 years.* Abstract 75, 1st World Congress of Hepato Pancreatico Biliary Surgery, Lund, June 1986.

27. Igawa S., Sakai K., Kinoshita H., Hirohashi K.: *Intraoperative sonography: clinical usefulness in liver surgery.* Radiology 156: 473–477, 1985.

28. Iwatsuki S., Shaw B., Starzl T.: *Experience with 150 liver resections.* Ann. Surg. 197: 247–253, 1983.

29. Johnson W. C., Gerzof S. G., Robbins A. N., Nabseth D. C.: *Treatment of abdominal abscess. Comparative evaluation of operative drainage guided by computed tomography or ultrasond.* Ann. Surg. 195: 510, 1981.

30. Karlson K. D., Martin E. C., Fankuchein, Schultz R. W., Caornella W. J.: *Percutaneous abscess drainage.* Surg. Gynecol. Obstet. 154: 44–47, 1982.

31. Kanematsu T., Takenada K., Matsumata T., Foruta T., Sugimachi K., Inokuschi K.: *Limited hepatic resection effective for selected cirrhotic patients with primary liver cancer.* Ann. Surg. 199: 51–56, 1984.

32. Kishi K., Shikate T., Hirohashi S. et al.: *Hepatocellular carcinoma, a clinical and pathological analysis of 57 hepatectomy cases.* Cancer 51: 542–548, 1983.

33. Landi F., Suraci V., Fianchini A.: *Il ruolo delle epatectomie maggiori nel trattamento delle metastasi epatiche da carcinoma colo-rettale.* In 'I tumori del fegato' G. Gozzetti et al., Editrice Compositori, Bologna, pp. 1985.

34. Lefkowitich J.H.: *The epidemiology and morphology of primary malignant liver tumors.* Surg. Clin. N. Amer. pp. 169–180, 1982.

35. Lim R. C., Bongard F. S.: *Hepatocellular carcinoma. Changing concepts in diagnosis and management.* Arch. Surg. 119, 637–641, 1984.

36. Lin T. Y., Lee C. S., Chen C. C. et al.: *Regeneration of human liver after hepatic lobectomy studied by repeated liver scanning and needle biopsy.* Ann. Surg. 190: 48–52, 1979.

37. Liver cancer study group of Japan: *Primary liver cancer in Japan.* Cancer 54: 1747–1755, 1984.

38. Machi J., Sigel B, Beitler J. C., Coelho J. C. U., Donahaue P. E., Duarte B., Nyhus L. M.: *Ultrasonic examination during surgery for abdominal abscess.* World J. Surg. 7: 409–415, 1983.

39. Makuuchi M., Hasegawa H., Yamasaki S.: *Intraoperative ultrasonic examination for hepatectomy.* Jpn. J. Clin. Oncol. 11, 367, 1981.

40. Makuuchi M., Hasegawa H., Yamasaki S. et al.: *Differences in clinicopathological features and clinical diagnosis of small hepatocellular carcinoma among each diameters less than 5 cm and it's treatment.* Acta Haptol. Jpn. 24: 1466–1468, 1983.
41. Makuuchi M., Hasegawa H., Yamasaki S.: *Ultrasonically guided subsegmentectomy.* Surg. Gynecol. Obstet. 161: 346–350, 1985.
42. Makuuchi M.: *Abdominal Intraoperative Ultrasonography.* Igaku-Shoin Ed., Tokyo, 1987.
43. Marchal G. J. F., Pylyser K., Tshibwabwa-Tumba E. et al.: *Anechoic halo in solid liver tumors: sonographic, microangiographic and histologic correlation.* Radiology 156: 479–484, 1985.
44. Nagasue N., Suehio S., Yakaya H.: *Intraoperative ultrasonography in the surgical treatment of hepatic tumors.* Acta Chir. Scand. 150: 311–316, 1984.
45. Nagasue N., Akamizu H., Yukaya H., Yunhi I.: *Hepatocellular pseudotumors in the cirrhotic liver.* Cancer 54: 2487–2494, 1984.
46. S., Okita M.: *Segmental and subsegmental resections of the cirrhotic liver under hepatic inflow and outflow occlusion.* Br. J. Surg. 72: 565–570, 1985.
47. Okamoto E., Tanaka N., Yamanaka N., Toyasaka A.: *Results of surgical treatment of primary hepatocellular carcinoma: some aspects to improve long term survival.* World J. Surg. 8: 360–366, 1984.
48. Okuda K., Musha H. et al.: *Clinicopathologic features of encapsuled hepatocellular carcinoma.* Cancer 40: 1240–1245, 1977.
49. Okuda K., Peters R., Sinson I.W.: *Gross anatomic features of hepatocellular carcinoma from three disparate geographic areas.* Cancer 54: 2165–2173, 1984.
50. Okuda K., Obate H., Nakajama Y., Ohtsuki T., Ohnishi K.: *Prognosis of primary hepatocellular carcinoma.* Hepatology 4 (S): 3–6, 1984.
51. Okuda K.: *What is the precancerous lesion for hepatocellular carcinoma in man?* J. Gastroenterol. Hepatol. 1: 79–85, 1986.
52. Possati L., Cavallari A., Gozzetti G., Mazziotti A., Bellusci R.: *'La chirurgia del fegato'* Masson Italia Ed., Milano, 1982.
53. Rubaltelli L., Del Maschio A., Cambiani F., Miotto D.: *The role of vascularization in the formation of echographic patterns of hepatic metastases: microangiographic and echographic study.* Br. J. Radiol. 53: 1166, 1980.
54. Sheu J. C., Sung J. L., Chen D. S., Yu J. Y., Wang T. H., Su C.T., Tsang Y. M.: *Ultrasonography of small hepatic tumors using high resolution linear array real time instruments.* Radiology 150: 797–802, 1984.
55. Sheu J. C., Lee C. S., Sung J. L., Chen D. S., Yang P. M., Lin T.Y.: *Intraoperative hepatic ultrasonography. An indispensable procedure in resection of small hepatocellular carcinoma.* Surgery 97: 97–103, 1985.
56. Shinagawa T., Ohto M., Okuda K.: *Diagnosis and clinical features of small hepatocellular carcinoma with emphasis on the utility of real-time ultrasonography.* Gastroenterology 86: 495–502, 1984.
57. Smith T. J., Kemeny M., Sugarbaker P. H., Jones A. E., Vermess M., Shawker T. N., Edwards B. K.: *A prospective study of hepatic imaging in the detection of metastatic disease.* Ann. Surg. 195: 486–491, 1982.
58. Subramanyan B. R., Balthazar E. J., Hilton S., Lefleur R. S., Horii S. C., Raghvendra B. N.: *Hepatocellular carcinoma with venous invasion: sonographic-angiographic correlation.* Radiology 150: 793–799, 1984.
59. Tagliacozzo S., Daniele G.M., Pisano G.: *Pericistectomia totale per echinococcosi del fegato.* Atti Soc. I. Chir. vol. I, C.L.U.E.B. Ed Bologna, 1979.
60. Tang Zhao-You: *Subclinical hepatocellular carcinoma.* Springer-Verlag, Berlin, 1985.
61. Tobe T.: *Hepatectomy in patients with cirrhotic livers: clinical and basic observations.* Surg. Annual (C.M. Nyhus Ed.): 177–202, 1984.
62. Ton That Tung: *Les résections majeures et mineures du foie.* Masson Ed., Paris, 1979.
63. Traynor O., Castaing D., Bismuth H.: *Peroperative ultrasonography in the surgery of hepatic tumors.* Br. J. Surg. 75: 197–202, 1988.

64. Trastek U. G., Van Heerden J. A., Sheedy P. F., Adson M. P.: *Cavernous hemangioma of the liver. Resect or observe?* Am. J. Surg. 145: 49–53, 1983.
65. Viscomi G. N., Gonzalez R., Taylor K. J.: *Histopathological correlation of ultrasound appearances of liver metastasis.* J. Clin. Gastroenterol. 3: 395–400, 1981.
66. Yamasaki S., Makuuchi M., Hasegawa H.: *Hepatic trisegmentectomy for liver cancer.* YRYO 36: 643, 1982.

Chapter 5: Intraoperative ultrasound during bile tract surgery

One of the first applications of intraoperative ultrasound, utilizing a compound scanner, was the investigation of the bile tract for the detection of stones [15, 28]. With the advent of real-time equipment, the main bile duct can be readily examined intraoperatively [5, 12, 26, 29, 30, 35, 38, 39, 42, 43, 44, 51], so much so that in many centers ultrasound represents a valid alternative to intraoperoperative cholangiography [26, 30, 46]. Furthermore, ultrasound has proved its usefulness during surgery for tumors of the porta hepatis and – a less frequent occurence – to repair post-operative stenosis.

Intraoperative exploration technique of the bile tree

Both gallbladder and the confluence of the hepatic ducts can be studied trans-hepatically placing a conventional transverse intraoperative probe on the 4th and 5th segments (Fig. 5.1). The common hepatic duct and the proximal two thirds of the gallbladder are readily visualized either by placing the probe directly on the bile tree or – by a trans-hepatic scan – resting the probe on Riedel's lobe on the sagittal plane, parallel to the lie of the gallbladder itself (Fig. 5.2). To visualize the distal third of the common bile duct and the papilla, the probe must rest directly either on the duodenum or the head of the pancreas, or directly on the common bile duct in a posterior approach, having mobilized the second portion of the duodenum. In our experience, razor-blade probes have proved useful since they can be placed on the lateral surface of the duodenum without having to detach this from the pancreas (Fig. 5.3). However, to be complete, an ultrasound picture must include visualization of the papilla.

Scanning can be performed on opening the abdomen, once the anterior surface of the liver is cleared of any adhesions due to previous surgery. Preliminary dissection of the hepatic peduncle is not necessary. Ultrasound investigation to ensure that a bile duct has been unplugged is not, however, practicable once the biliary tree has been opened since the presence of air bubbles causes high-level echoes that throw up acoustic shadows. Similarly, US scan is not feasible following transcystic cholangiography.

Bile tree anatomy at ultrasound

The common bile duct appears as an anechoic tubular structure, parallel and

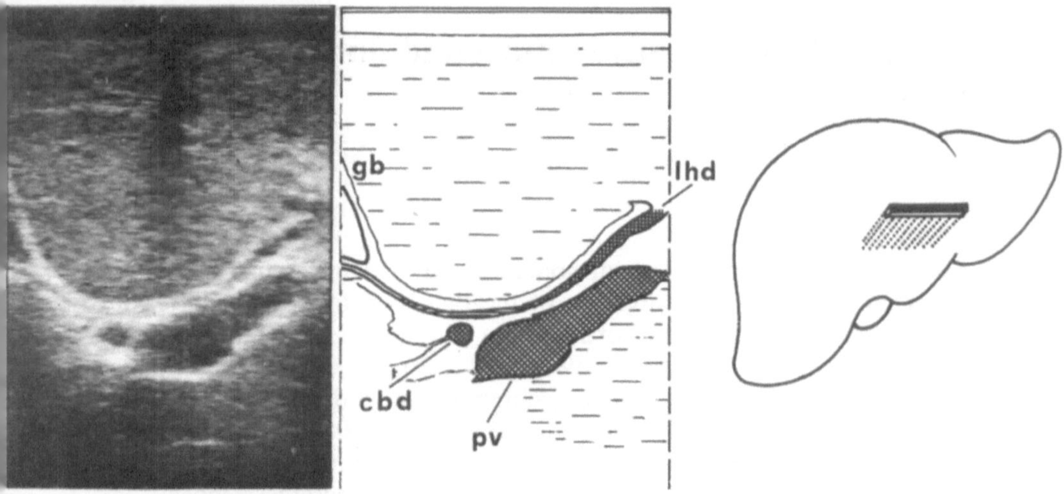

A

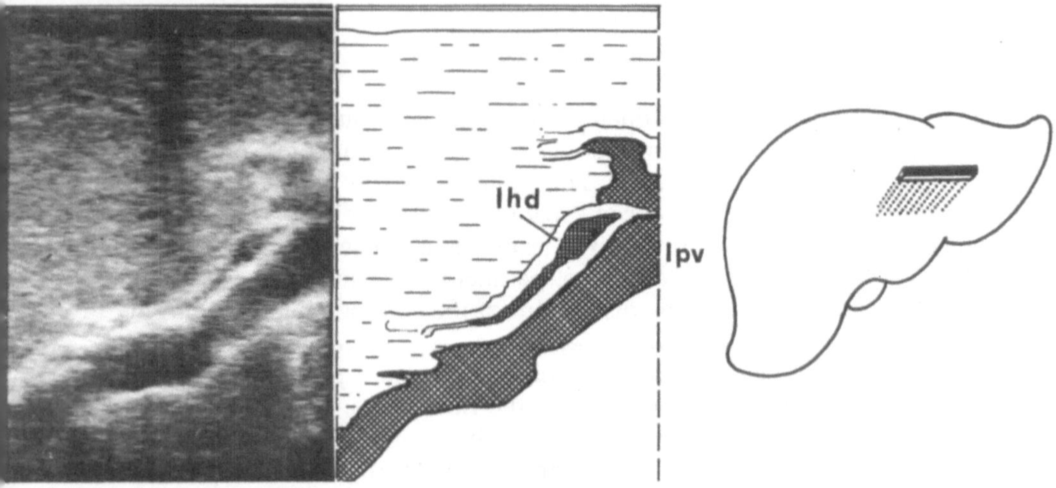

gb

lhd

cbd

pv

B

lhd

lpv

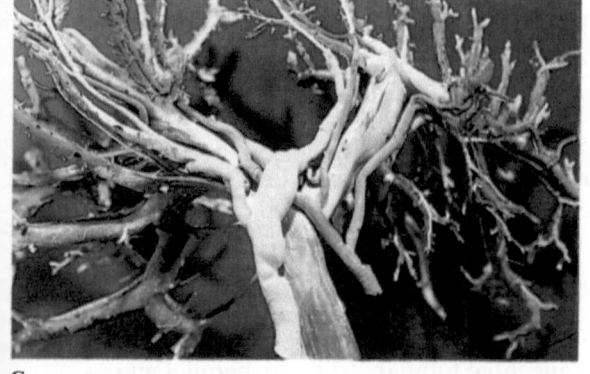

C

Figure 5.1.

A) *Porta hepatis* seen on transverse sc
through the 4th segment. The fundus of t
gallbladder (gb) is visible, along with the con
mon bile duct (cbd), the portal bifurcatio
(pv) and the left hepatic duct (lhd); the ll
and the left branch of the portal vein are mo
clearly evidenced if the probe is shifted late
ally towards the left lobe (B).

C) A resin cast of the branches of the port
vein, hepatic artery and common bile duct
the porta hepatis.

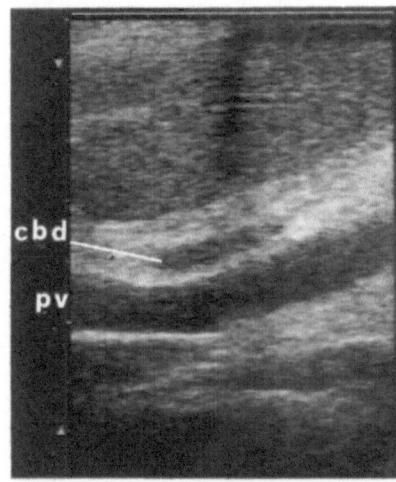

Figure 5.2. Common bile duct (cbd) on transhepatic scan with probe on the 4th segment on the sagittal plane. Note that the cbd is anterior to the portal vein (pv).

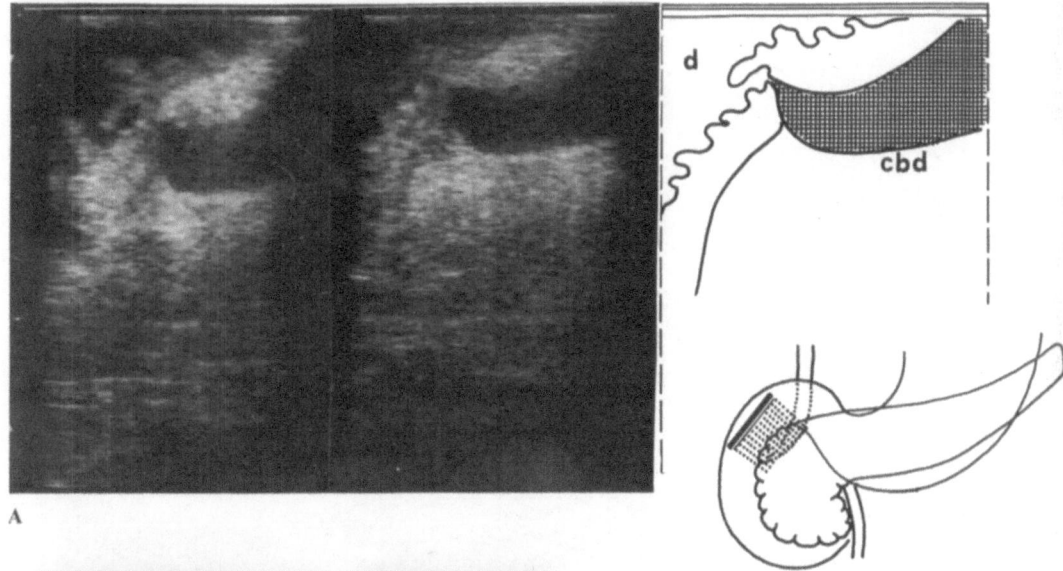

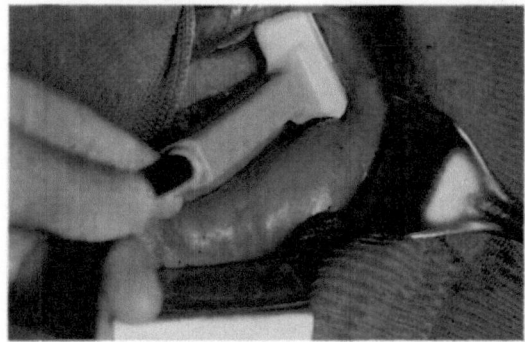

Figure 5.3. Distal end of the common bile duct. Longitudinal scan; the probe lies laterally on the distal portion of the common bile duct (A).

B) Although bile duct diameter is notably increased, there is no mechanical obstruction in the papillar region. (72 year old patient with sclero-atrophic gallbladder caused by stones). Cerulein was administered to induce filling of the duodenum with bile.

76

anterior to the portal vein. Its normal diameter ranges from 2–3 mm to 5–6 mm, with a tendency to increase with aging. In fact, in elderly or previously cholecystectomized patients or in the case of non-visualization of a sclero-atrophic gallbladder, the common bile duct may be markedly dilated. Ultrasound is particularly effective in identifying or ruling out the presence of stones in hydrops of the common bile duct. Moreover this examination affords a truly physiologic study of papilla patency and change of bile tract diameter following administration of cerulein (Fig. 5.4). Since the point of

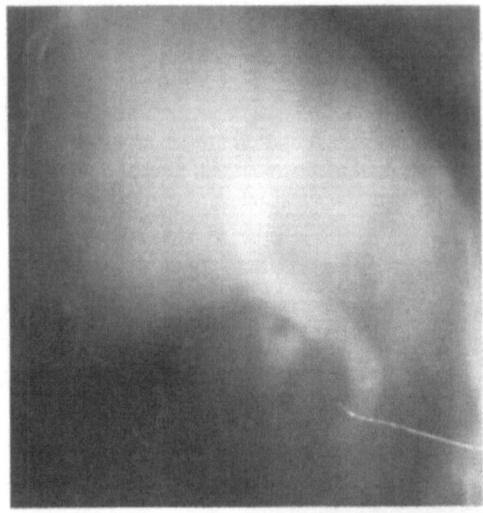

A

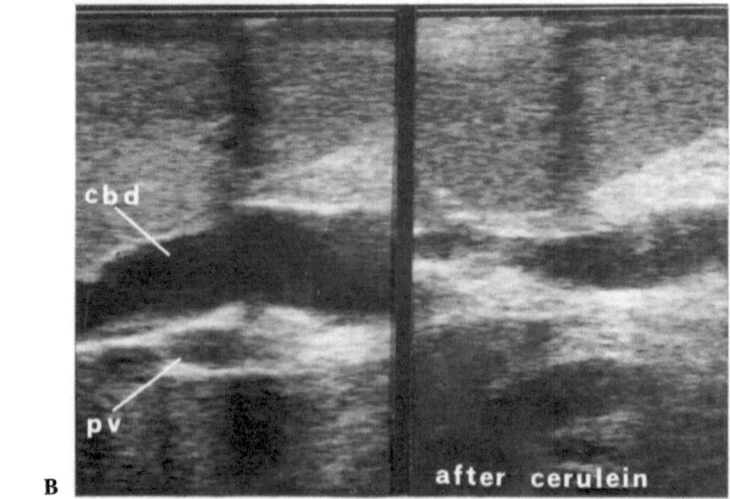

B

Figure 5.4. Same case as previous figure.
A) Preoperative cholangiography. Dilated hepatic duct and non-visualized galbladder.
B) Longitudinal scan on Riedel's lobe. Cerulein administration induces sharp reduction in bile duct diameter.

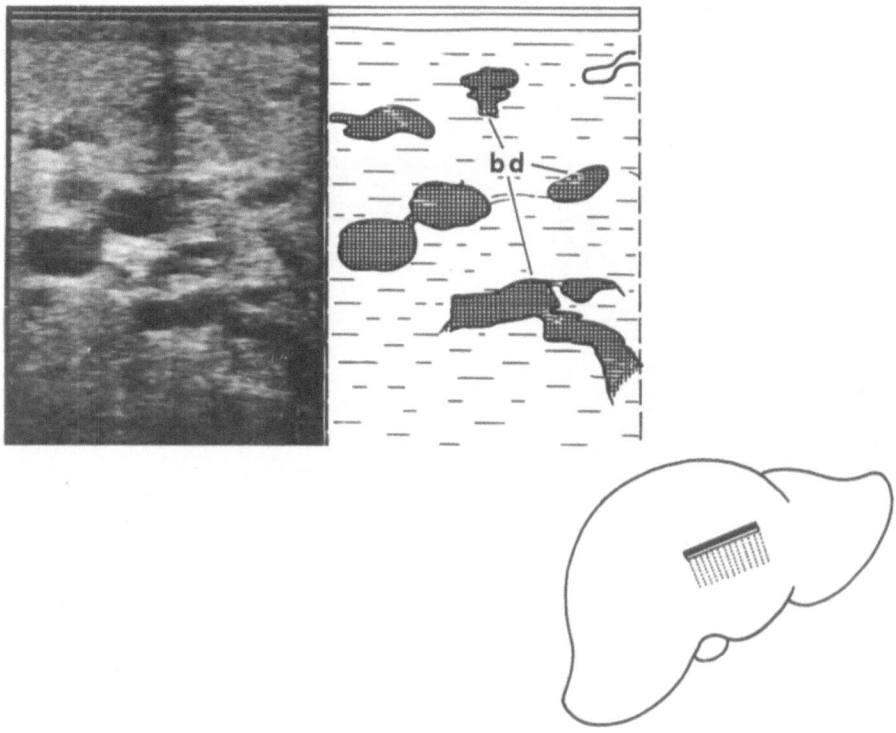

Figure 5.5. Dilation of the intrahepatic biliary tree due to ampullary neoplasm. Transverse scan on the right liver lobe.

entry of the papilla can be readily visualized, the passage of bile – typically dense and hypoechoic – can be followed into the duodenum.

Proceeding upwards, the cystic duct is then visualized along with any embedded stones. Then comes the bifurcation of the hepatic ducts above the portal branches, the left duct being longer and slightly larger than the right and running parallel to the left branch of the portal vein (Fig. 5.1).

Under normal conditions the intrahepatic biliary tract cannot be distinguished from the wall of the portal vessels. In case of obstruction, the intrahepatic bile ducts can de differentiated from the adjacent portal branches on account of the absence of blood flow. In Figure 5.5 the right hand side of the biliary tree appears tortuous while on the left, the ducts of the 2nd and 3rd segment are long, straight, parallel and, in places, larger than the portal vessels (Fig. 5.6). The ducts of these particular segments can be readily identified at intraoperative ultrasound, a considerable help when carrying out peripheral cholangio-jejunal anastomoses.

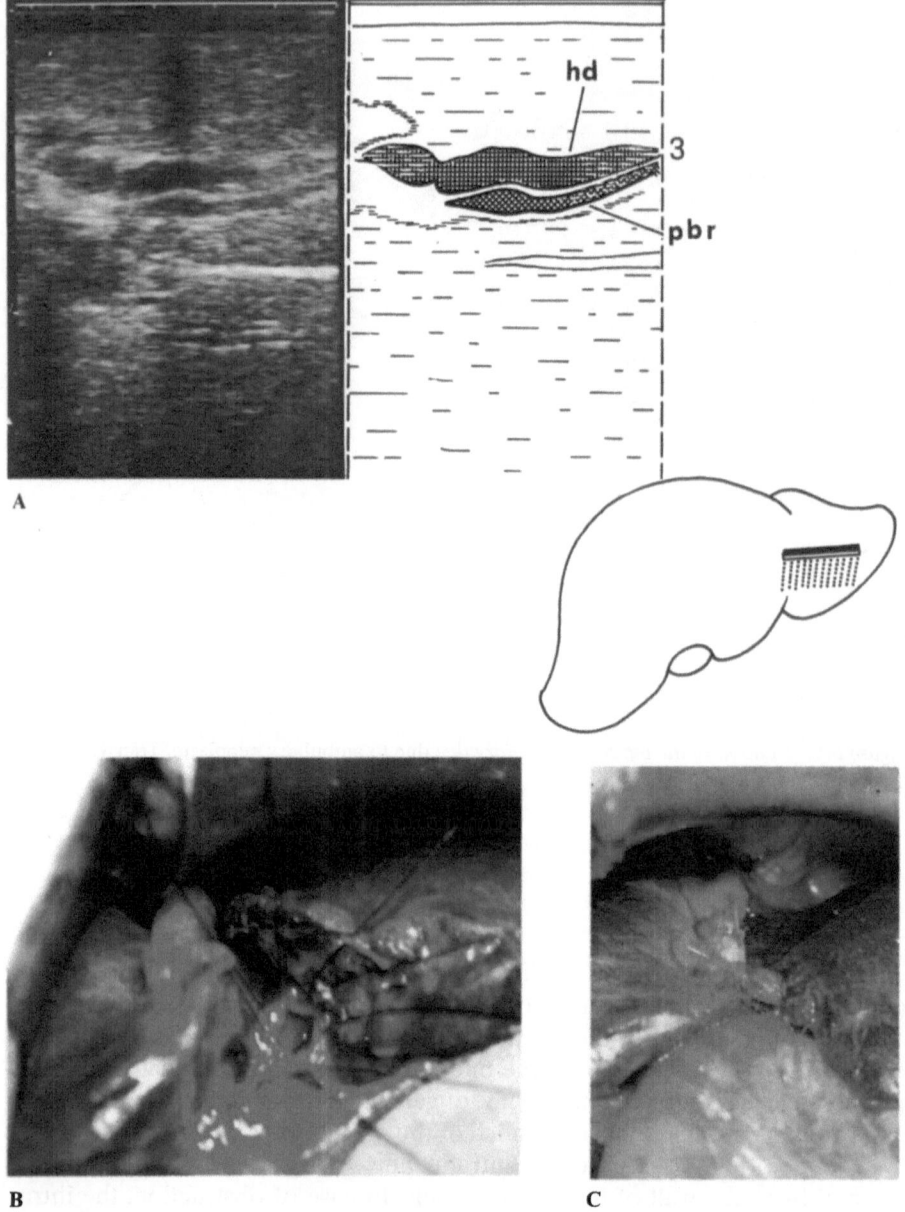

Figure 5.6.
A) *Dilatation of the left side of the billiary tree.*
Being able to identify the duct in the 3rd segment is of considerable practical help when performing palliative cholangio-jejunal anastomosis, in this case for bile duct tumor at the porta hepatis.
B) Duct in the 3rd segment subsequent to incision of the liver along the plane of the falciform ligament as it enters the liver.
C) View of the cholangio-jejunal anastomosis.

Biliary stones

In *gallbladder disease* intraoperative ultrasound usually affords little additional information to trans-abdominal scan. There are a few exceptions, namely stones in cirrhotic (Fig. 5.7) and obese subjects [23], identification of polyps (Fig. 5.8) and more especially, very small stones in the gallbladder. Indeed *microlithiasis* is missed frequently at cholecystography and also occasionally at preoperative scan [10, 24] but can be clearly differentiated from bile sludge at intraoperative examination. Sludge develops due to bile stasis or prolonged fasting [8] and appears as homogeneous, weakly echogenic debris lying on the inferior wall of the gallbladder (Fig. 5.9). Minute stones, on the other hand, show up clearly as high-level echoes with a thin shadow which gives them an unmistakable appearance (Fig. 5.10). Stones as small as 1 millimeter can be detected.

Intraoperative ultrasound in bile surgery has its main application in the *diagnosis of stones in the main bile ducts*. As mentioned above, even small size stones are identified as well as bile altered by pus or sludge (Fig. 5.11). Stones give hyperechoic images casting acoustic shadows of an amplitude proportional to stone size (Fig. 5.12). However, as with trans-abdominal ultrasound, this posterior shadow is not a constant feature [13, 41]: soft or pigment stones, especially if small, are often highly echogenic without giving rise to any shadow. Moreover the shadow may be masked by the echo-spared area of a dilated biliary duct lumen [42]. However both the number and site of stones can be accurately determined for proximal calculi as well as stones impacted in the papilla (Fig. 5.13).

The condition par excellence in which ultrasonic investigation truly stands out is in the detection of *intrahepatic stones*. These may well escape detection at intraoperative cholangiography especially if the stones are peripheral [21],

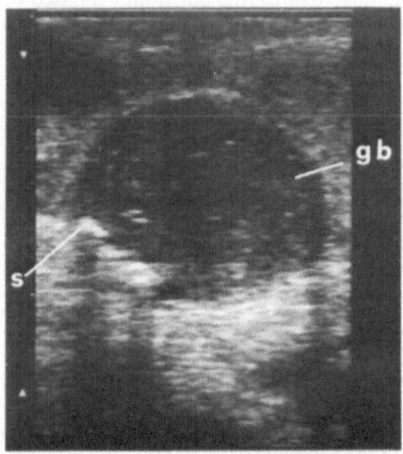

Figure 5.7. Gallstones in a cirrhotic patient. Dilated gallbladder filled with sludge.

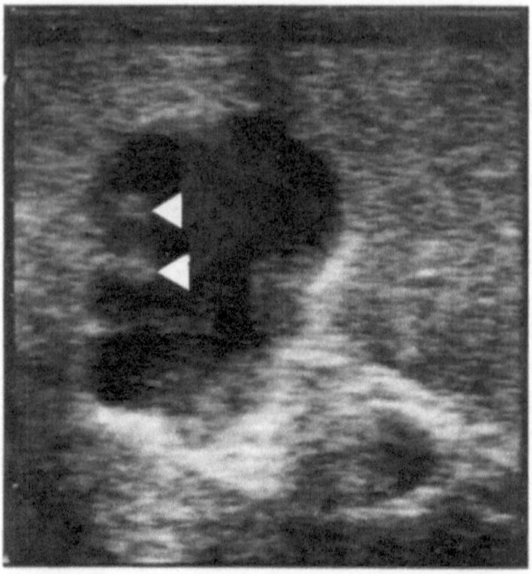

A

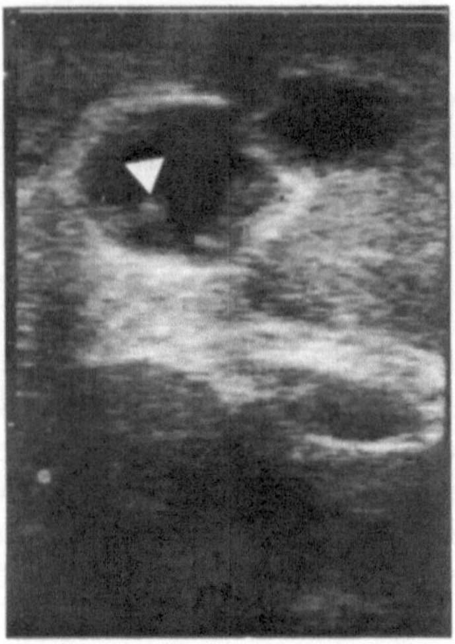

B

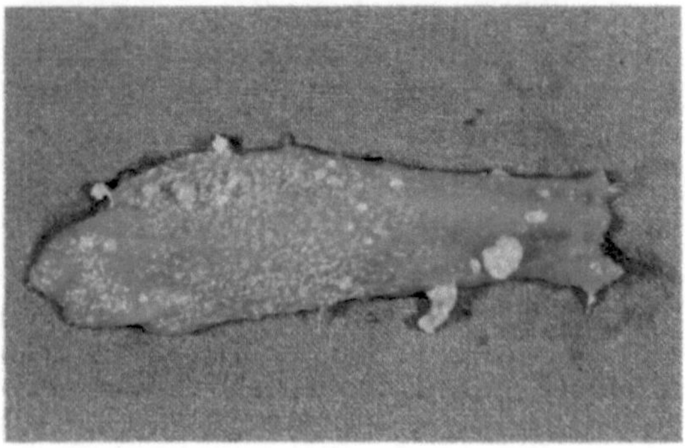

C

Figure 5.8. Cholesterolosis of the gallbladder. Numerous pedunculated polyps (arrow) project into the lumen. Differential diagnosis to rule out stones is based on the weaker echogenicity of polyps, their marked mobility and absence of back shadow. Longitudinal (A) and transverse scan (B) of the fundus. C) Surgical specimen.

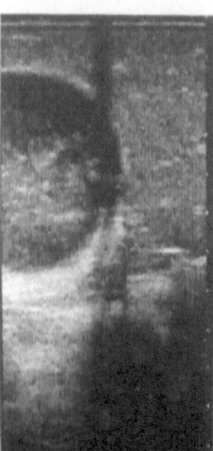

Figure 5.9. Billiary sludge in a distended gall-bladder in a patient with malignant growth of the head of the pancreas.

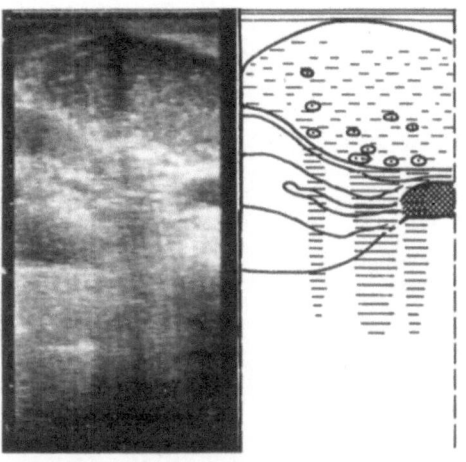 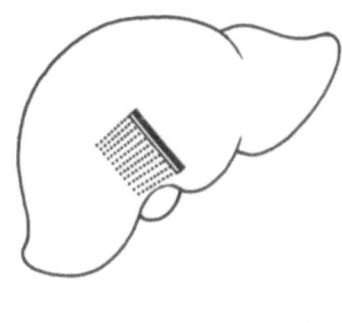

Figure 5.10. Microlithiasis of the gallbladder associated with biliary sludge. This female patient had presented recurrent episodes of acute pancreatitis; pre-operative cholangiography showed normal gallbladder. The very small stones appear as small blocks of high-level echoes lying along the lower wall of the gallbladder and casting fine acoustic shadows.

but return unmistakable echoes from within the parenchyma and adjacent to a portal branch. The bile duct may also appear dilated proximal to the stone (Fig. 5.14). Posterior shadow may or may not be present. Should the intra-hepatic stones be localized in the bile ducts of just one segment or sector of the liver, they pebble and even fill the whole bile duct segment, the lumen of which becomes indistinct. The extent of stone disease is readily assessed in these cases, providing valuable information for segmental resection [1] (Fig. 5.16).

Lane [30], Sigel [46] and Jakimowicz [27] have published prospective studies comparing the diagnostic accuracy of ultrasound with that of intra-operative cholangiography (Table 5.1). Lane reports similar sensitivity and

Table 5.1. Results of intraoperative ultrasonography and cholangiography in the diagnosis of choledocolithiasis

	Intraop. ultrasonography			Intraop. cholangiography		
	Lane (100 cases)	Sigel (350 cases)	Jakimowicz (383 cases)	Lane	Sigel	Jakimowicz
Sensitivity %	96	93.8	92.3	96	90.9	86.2
Specificity %	93	98.6	98.9	96	95.4	94.9
Accuracy %	–	98	94.9	–	94.8	89.2
Positive pre-dictive value	–	91	96.5	–	73.2	95.6
Negative pre-dictive value	–	99	97	–	98.7	96

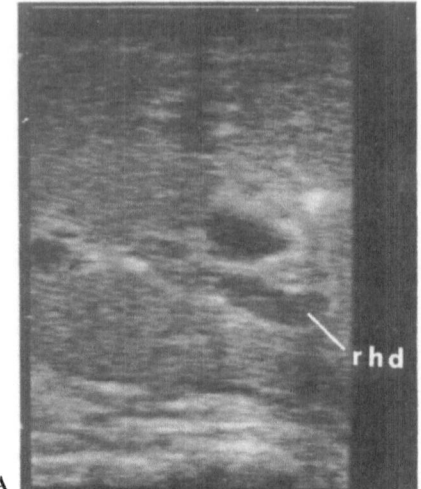

A

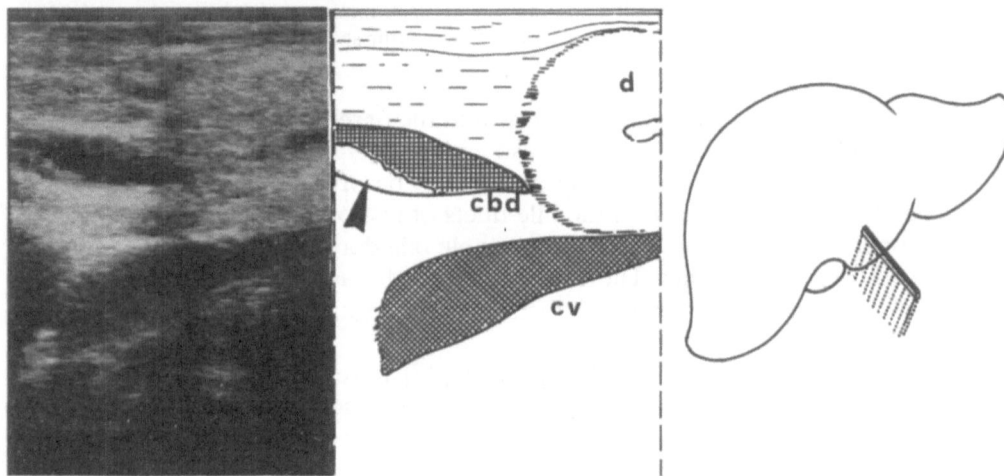

B

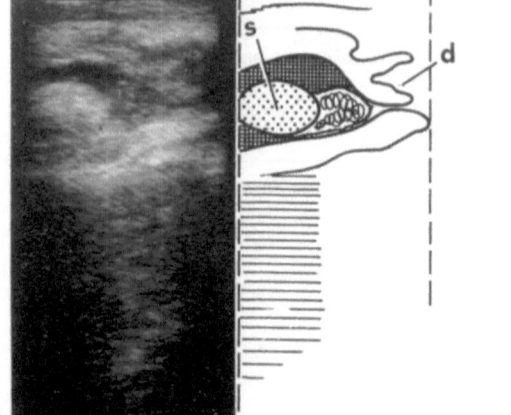

C

Figure 5.11. Sludge in the biliary tree.
A) In the right hepatic duct.
B) In the distal common bile duct.
C) Associated with an iuxta-papillary stone(s).

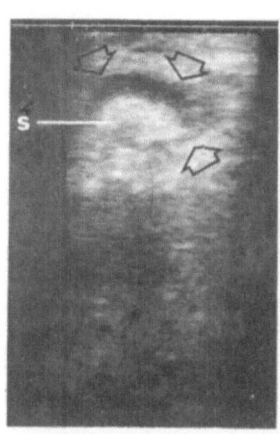
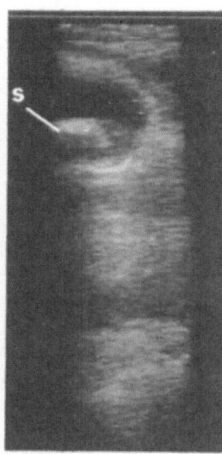

Figure 5.12. Stones in the common bile duct.
A, B, C) Direct contact scans on the biliary
tract. The main bile duct appears dilated with
stones (s) that project a posterior shadow.
Transhepatic scan.
D) Large stone in the proximal common bile
duct with shadow.

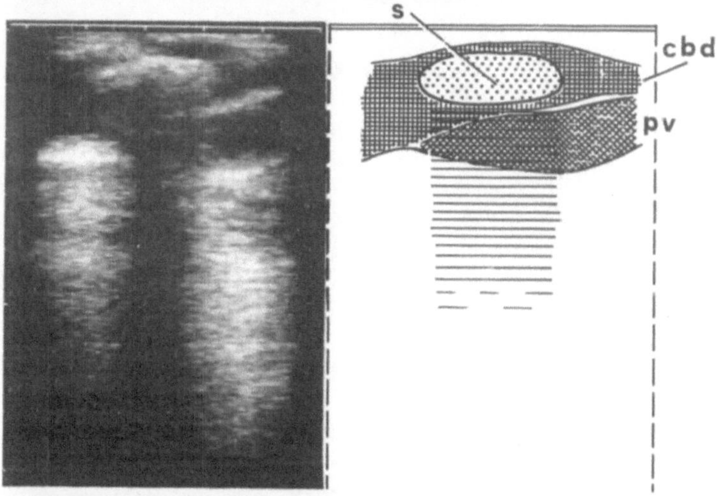

A

B

C

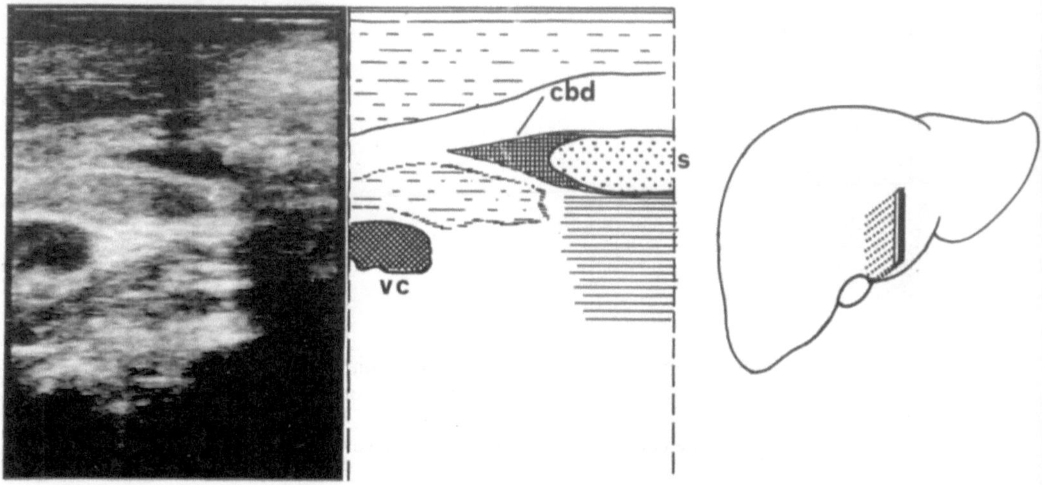

D

84

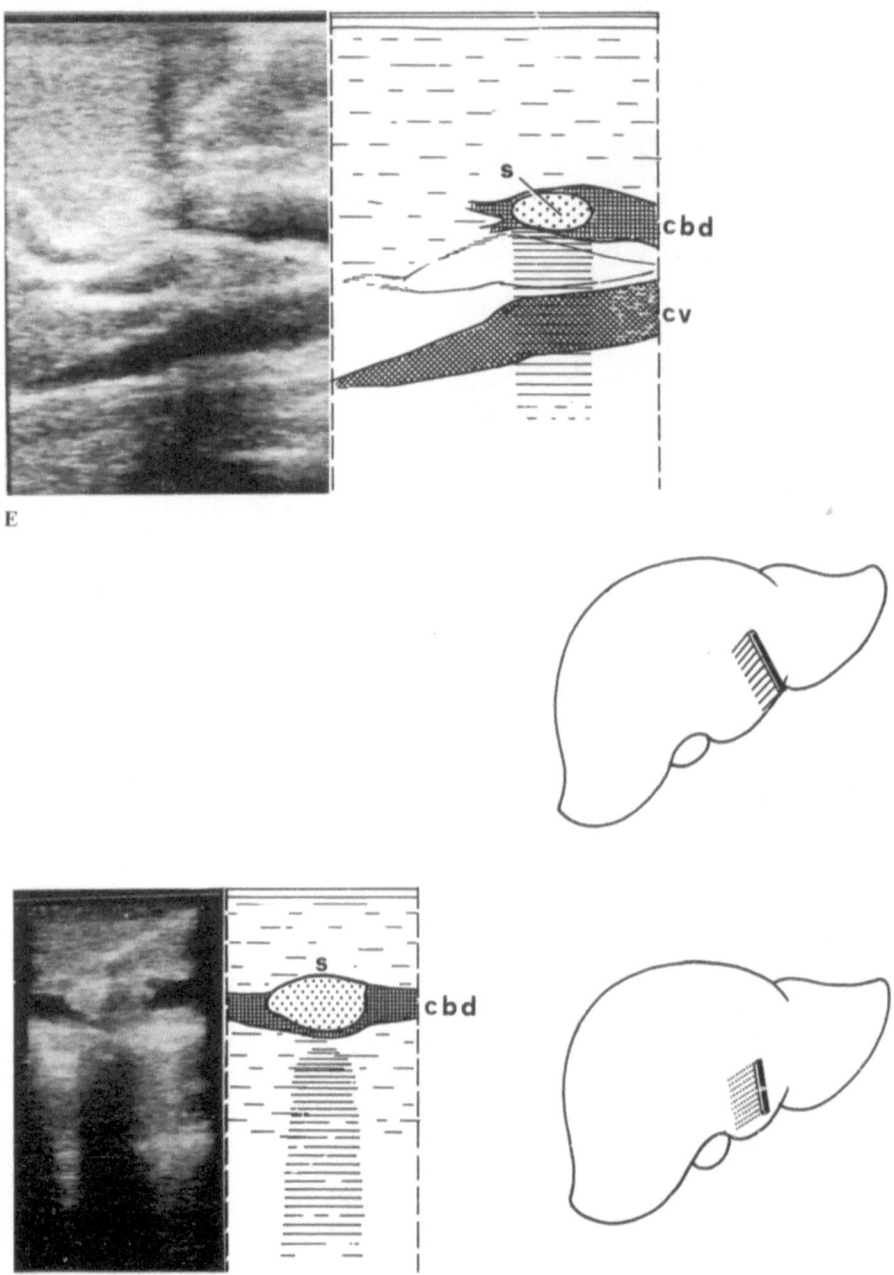

E

F

Figure 5.12. Stones in the common bile duct (case study continued).
E) As in the previous case, the stone is in the proximal common bile duct but the shadow is less evident.
F) Longitudinal scan of the common bile duct. Here too a voluminous stone is visible with an evident shadow.

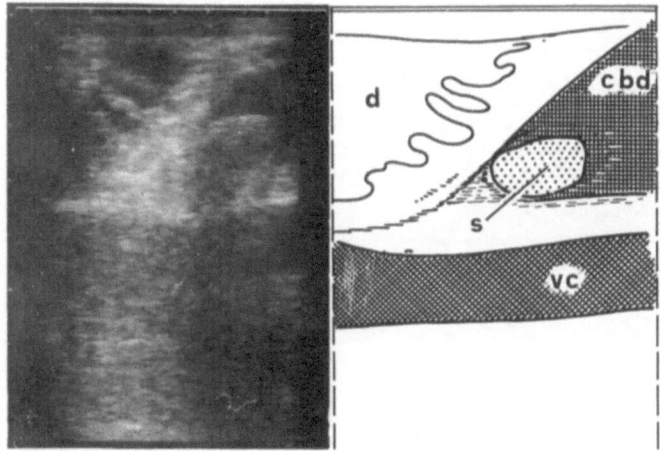

Figure 5.13. Stone embedded in the papilla of vater. The bile duct proximal to the calculus is evidently dilated.

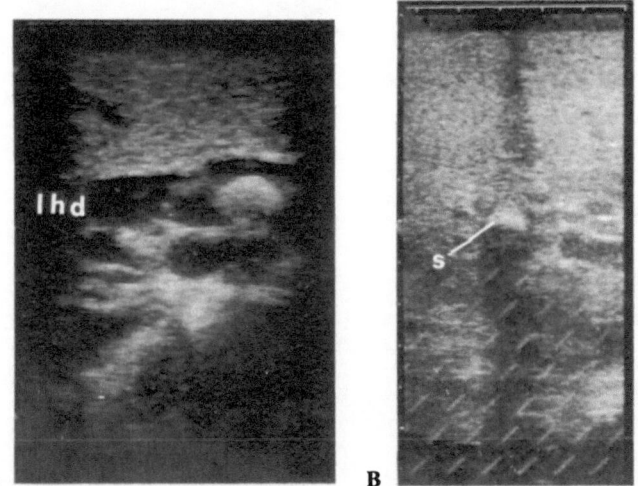

A   **B**

Figure 5.14. Intrahepatic lithiasis.
A) Calculus in the left hepatic duct (lhd). Transverse scan on the left lobe.
B) Calculus (s) in the right hepatic duct with evident shadow.

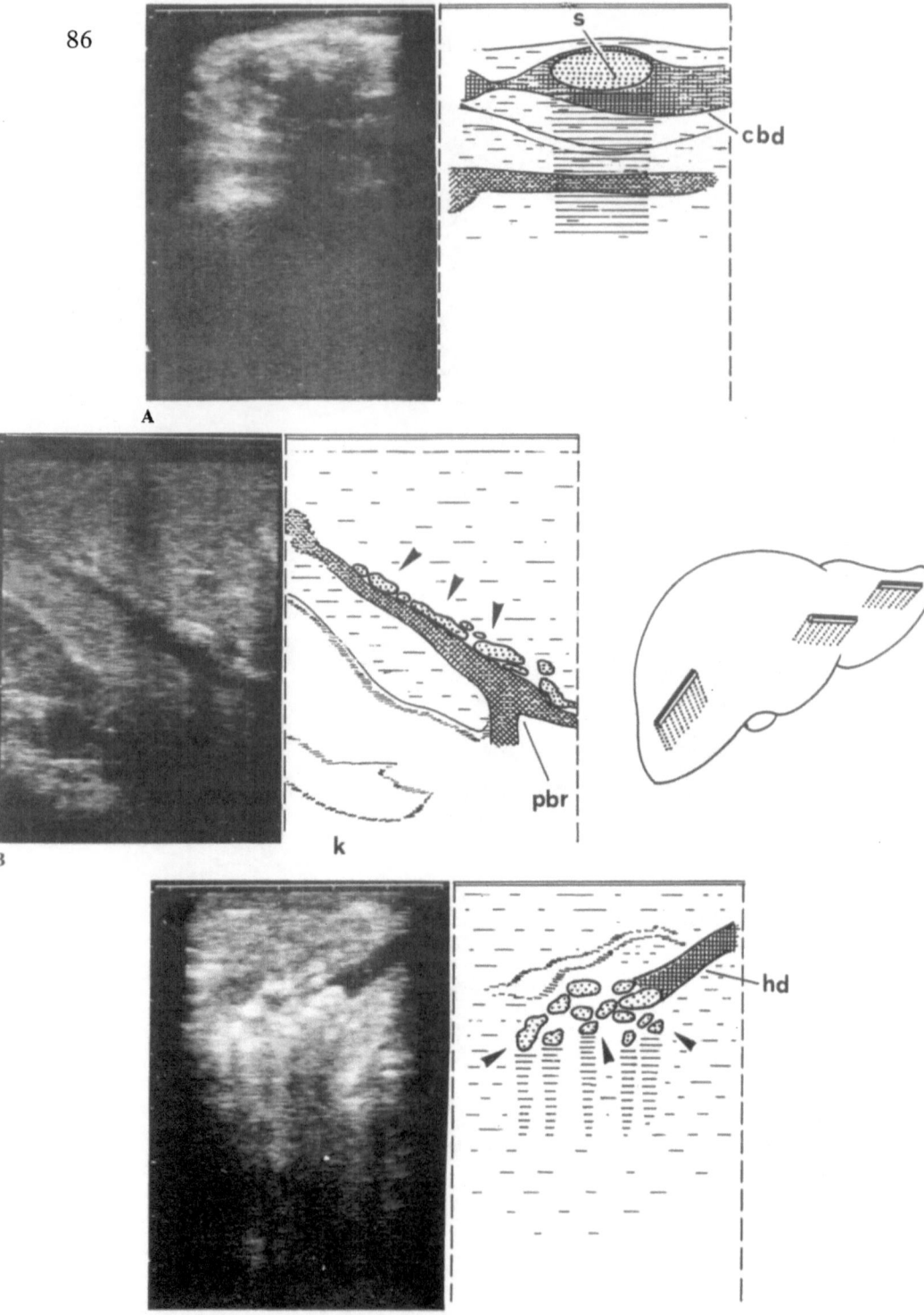

Figure 5.15. Intra-hepatic stones. Patient with multiple common bile duct stones (A). Scans of segment 6 (B) and 4 (C) show many small stones, some of which casting acoustic shadows, in the intrahepatic bile ducts. In C the proximal bile duct appear dilated. A Roux loop with hepatic jejunostomy was performed.

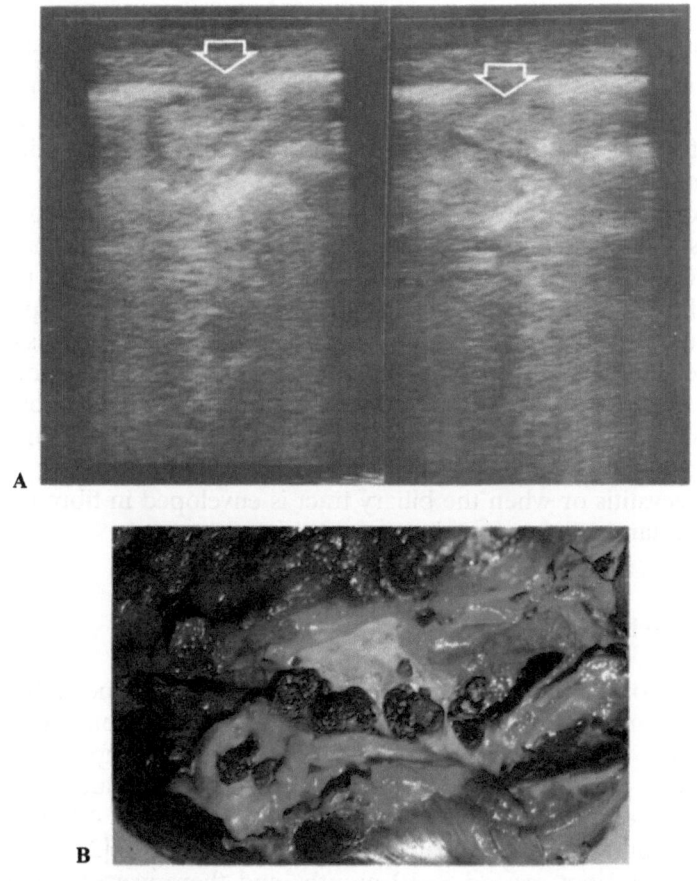

Figure 5.16. Intra-hepatic stones.
A) Several large echogenic stones (arrow) without back shadow occupy the entire lumen of the hepatic ducts of the 3th segment. Air in the upper part of the bile duct is visible as a hyper-echoic band returning reverberations. Surgery consisted of left lobectomy (B).

specificity for both methods while Sigel indicates ultrasound as being both more reliable and easier to perform as well as more economic than cholangiography. As a result, ultrasound is considered the method of choice for the screening of stones in the main bile tract [46]. More recently, Jakimowicz's data not only further confirm the usefulness of intraoperative ultrasound in screening for common duct stones, but moreover attribute greater specificity and predictive value to positive findings by u.s. compared to cholangiography, i.e. that there is a lower probability of false positives with the use of ultrasound. The author concludes that ultrasound may in future become a valid alternative to routine cholangiography [27].

These data have still to be corroborated by further studies and the cholangiography in question may not have been performed under the best possible conditions (use of only standard radiograms; manual injection without the aid of a radiomanometer). We believe that ultrasound and cholangiography cannot be considered alternative methods since intraoperative cholangiography is mandatory during bile tract surgery, supplying as it does capital information on the anatomy of the intra and extra-hepatic bile tree and the functional capacity of the papilla.

Radiological images are certainly more objective and less dependent on operator skill and technical excellence as are ultrasound techniques. The two methods would therefore seem complementary, with ultrasound proving its worth in those circumstances in which intraoperative cholangiography is most likely to suffer from an error of interpretation, in the event of gross dilatation of the bile duct [11, 15] or when there is greater likelihood of intrahepatic stones in a patient with multiple lithiasis [21], or in cases of intolerance or hypersensitivity to contrast medium [35]. There are the circumstances in which transcystic cholangiography is not technically practicable, such as in acute cholecystitis or when the biliary tract is enveloped in fibrous scar secondary to inflammation or previous surgery.

Tumors of the biliary tree

Management of tumors of the biliary tree, especially at the porta hepatis, is a technically complex problem and still a matter of some controversy. In the past, palliative procedures were very common in an attempt to resolve the accompanying jaundice: hepatic-jejunal diversions on the duct of the 3rd or even 5th segment in the case of proximal tumors [4, 7, 14, 40, 47] or, as an alternative, trans-tumoral intubation with silastic catheters [25, 37, 48]. As a rule survival did not exceed 8–10 months and there were frequent angiocolitic complications [36]. Recently a more aggressive approach consisting of tumor ablation has been advocated for these malignancies as well, since in carefully selected patients this has been reported to give better chances of survival, fewer complications and a better quality of life [2, 3, 6, 10, 17, 18, 20, 22, 32, 33, 34, 36, 49, 50, 52]. In fact this type of tumor is usually circumscribed, with hepatic or lymph node metastases appearing only much later on, especially in the case of so-called Klatskin tumors which form at the confluence of the bile ducts. Resection is therefore indicated for these forms of localized tumors with no hepatic or lymph node involvement or infiltration of the portal bifurcation. Several resection procedures have been proposed depending on the hepatic or intraductal extension of the tumor, i.e. resection of the confluence of the bile ducts and ablation of part of the liver parenchyma, followed by double cholangio-jejunal anastomosis onto the left and right hepatic duct [22] or left or right hepatectomy if only one side of the biliary tree is involved, with cholangio-jejunal anastomosis; on occasion a segment of portal vein may also have to be removed if found to be invaded by tumor [18, 34, 50].

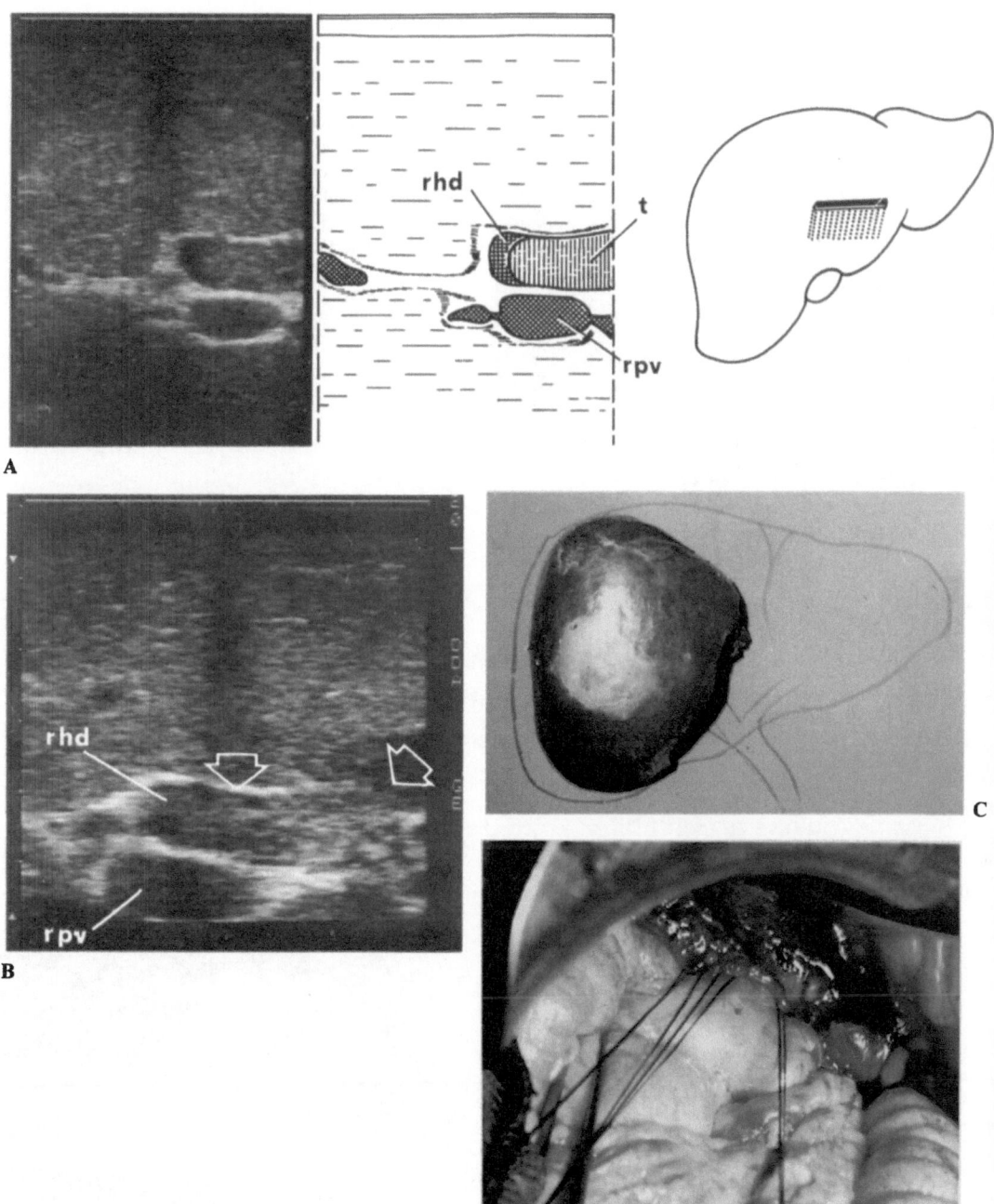

Figure 5.17. Neoplasia in the right hepatic duct.
The tumor occupies the whole of the duct lumen (A), extending from the bifurcation to second-ary branches. Right hepatectomy (C) was performed with cholangio-jejunal anastomosis onto the left hepatic duct (D).

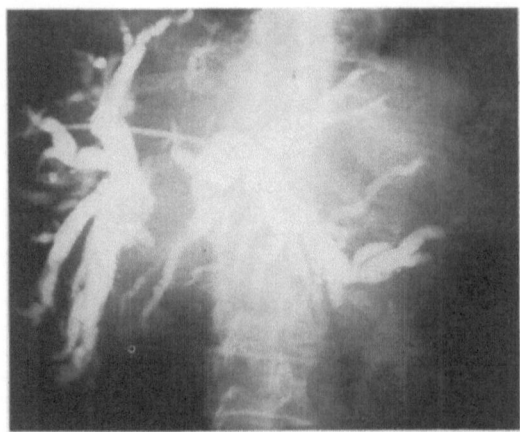

A

Figure 5.18. Klatskin tumor.

A) Transhepatic cholangiography shows obstruction of the confluence of the bile ducts.

B) Intraoperative ultrasound shows the tumor as a prevalently hyperchoic yet irregular mass anterior to the portal bifurcation. The proximal bile ducts are clearly dilated.

A wedge resection including the bifurcation (C) was carried out with double anastomosis of the left and right hepatic duct onto an isolated loop (D).

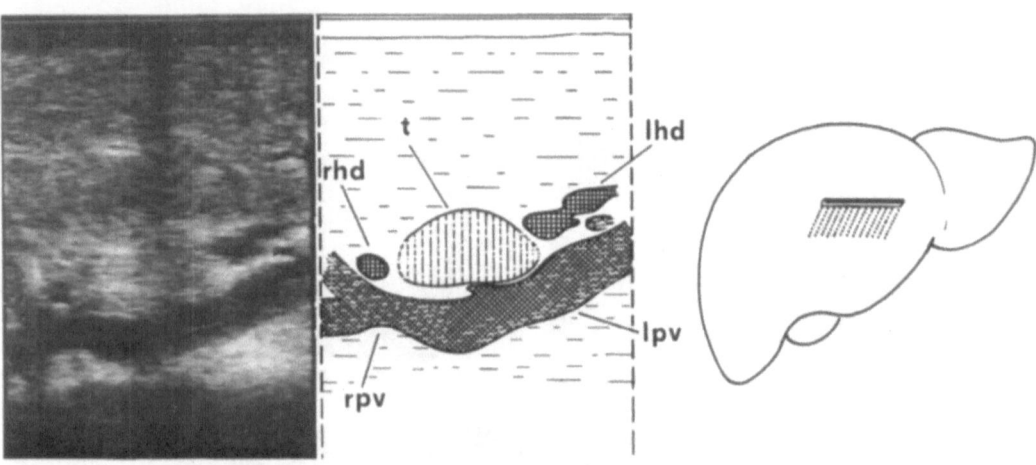

B

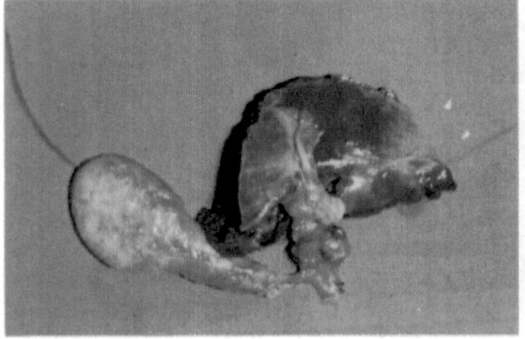

C

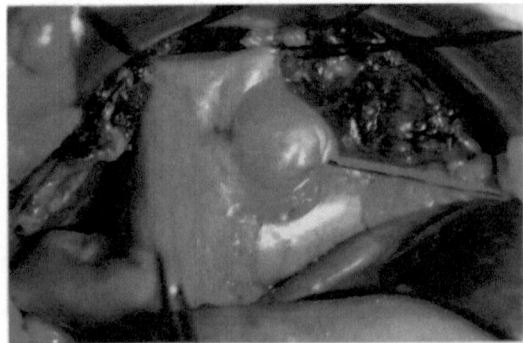

D

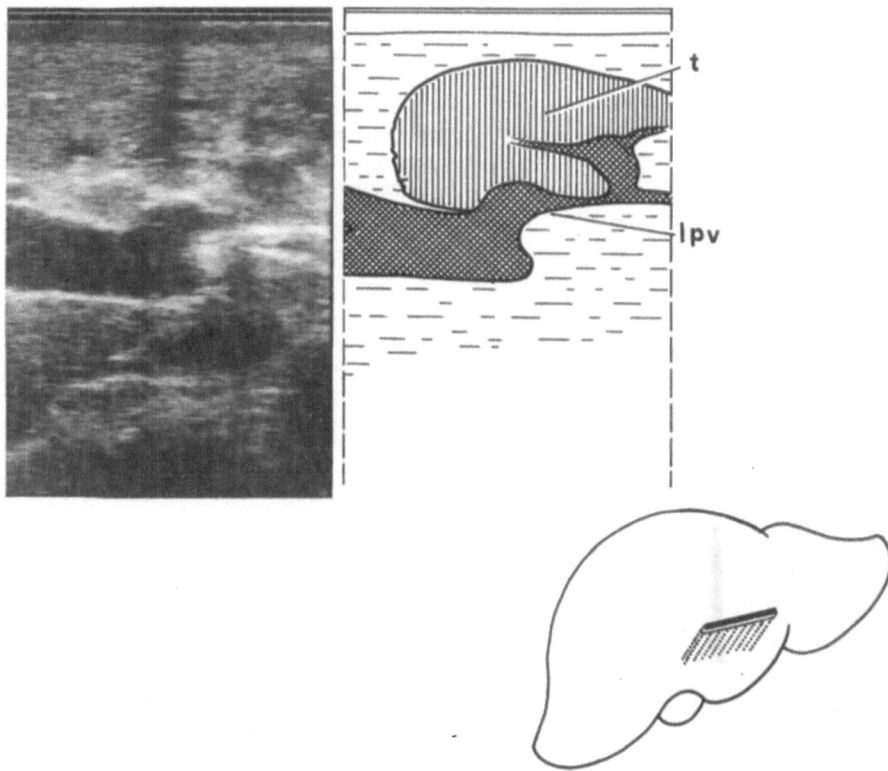

Figure 5.19. Tumor of the left hepatic duct with infiltration of the liver parenchyma.
The appearance of the lesion is irregular and poorly marginated.

While cholangiography and pre-operative ultrasound show only indirect signs of neoplasia in the form of biliary tree obstruction, intraoperative ultrasound allows visualization of the lesion itself. This appears in the bile duct as a solid mass of low-level echoes with poorly defined contours (Fig. 5.17). The actual wall of the bile ducts may be breached or totally unrecognizable on account of tumor infiltration (Fig. 5.18). When the tumor has reached the liver parenchyma its margins become difficult to distinguish (Fig. 5.19) and only rarely does one see a well circumscribed mass (Fig. 5.20). Indeed this tendency to infiltrate and hence return ill-defined images is the main reason why pre-operative ultrasound and CT scanning fail to detect the lesion [36]. Intraoperative ultrasound, however, can pinpoint infiltration of the portal bifurcation, evidenced by the disappearance of the high-level echoes returned by the vein wall or the presence of an intraluminal neoplastic thrombus (Fig. 5.21). Furthermore, as this examination is especially helpful in indicating the extent of local as well as metastatic disease, it proves of capital importance to the surgeon. In palliative surgery, ultrasound is all-important in identifying the bile ducts for peripheral intrahepatic bilio-digestive anastomosis and in guiding the drainage catheters to the correct position.

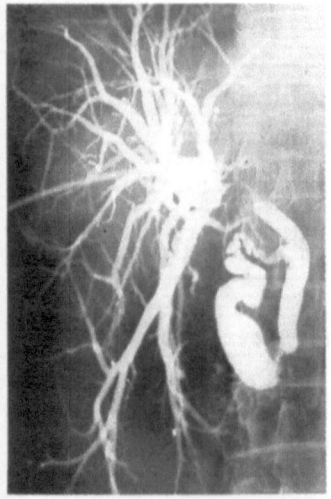

Figure 5.20. Neoplasm of the confluence of the bile ducts.
A) Transhepatic cholangiography shows an obstruction of the confluence. At intraoperative ultrasound the tumor appears as an echogenic area extending beyond the bile duct into the caudate lobe (B, C).

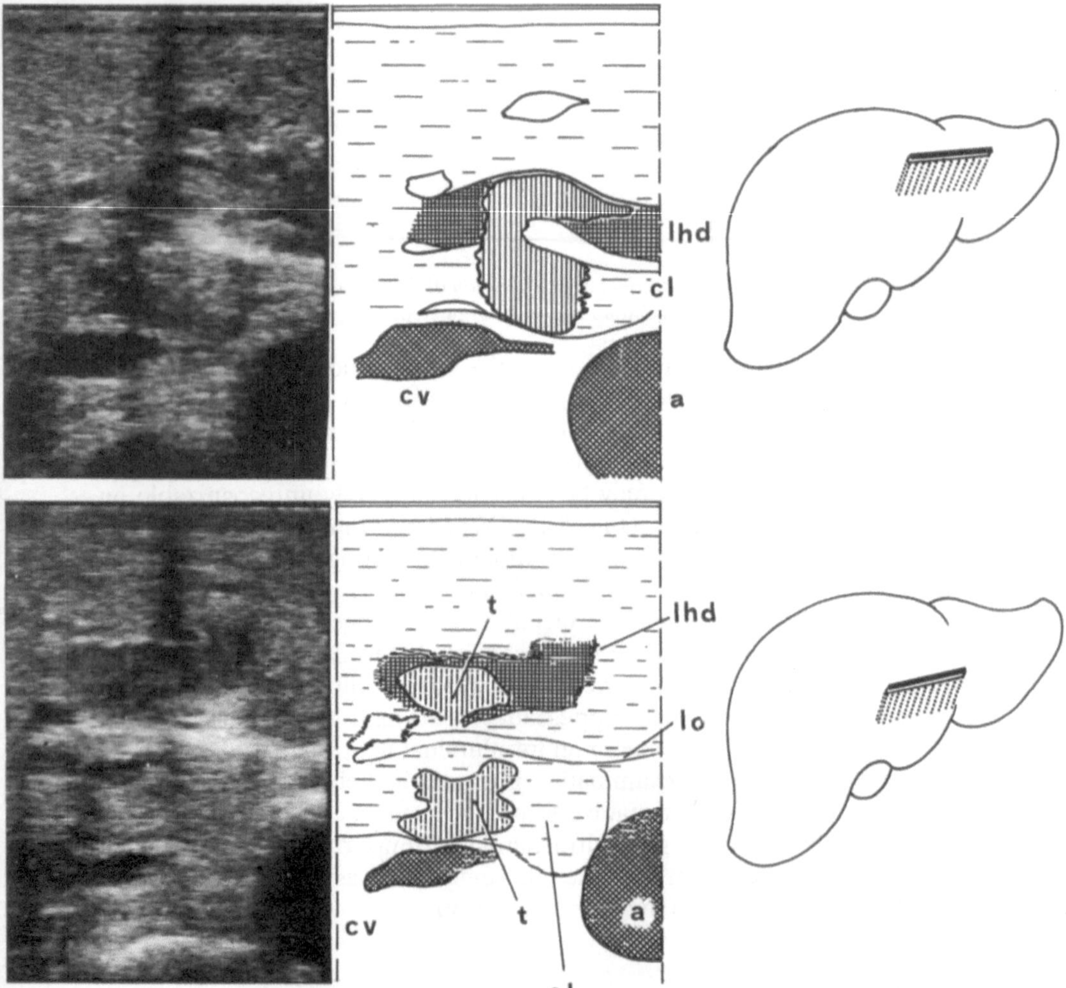

lhd

cl

cv

a

t

lhd

lo

cv

t

a

cl

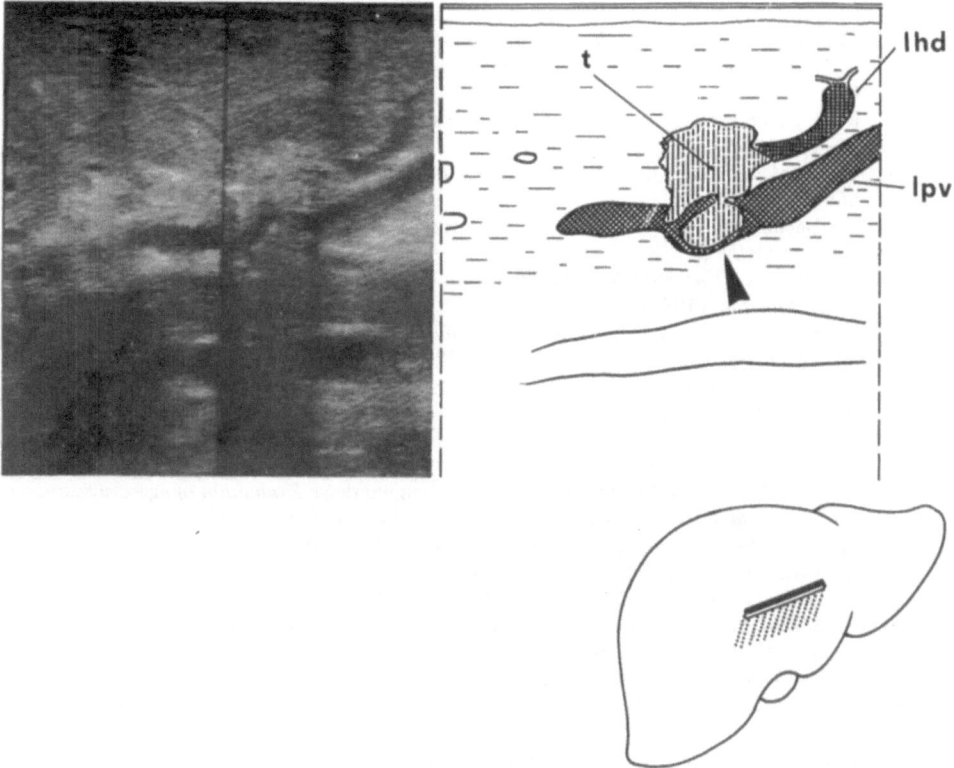

Figure 5.21. Klatskin tumor (t) with neoplastic thrombosis (arrow) of the portal birfurcation.

References

1. Adson M. A., Nagorney D. M.: *Hepatic resections for intrahepatic ductal stones.* Arch. Surg. 117: 611–161, 1982.
2. Beazley R. M., Hadjis N., Benjamin I. S. et al.: *Clinicopathological aspects of high bile duct cancer: experience with resection and bypass surgical treatment.* Ann. Surg. 199: 623–636, 1984.
3. Bengmark S., Ekberg H., Klofver-Stahl B., Evander A., Tranberg K. G.: *Long term survival after major liver resection for Klatskin tumor.* Abstract 283, 1st World Congress of Hepato-Pancreatico-Biliary Surgery, Lund, June 1986.
4. Bismuth H., Corlette M. B.: *Intrahepatic cholangioenteric anastomosis in carcinoma of the hilus of the liver.* Surg. Gynecol. Obstet. 140: 170–8, 1975.
5. Bismuth H., Castaing D., Kunstilnger F.: *L'echographie per-opératoire en chirurgie hépato-biliaire.* Presse Méd. 13: 1819–1822, 1984.
6. Blumgart L. H., Hadjis N. S., Benjamin I. S., Beazley R.: *Surgical approaches to cholangio-carcinoma at confluence of hepatic ducts.* Lancet 1: 66–70, 1984.
7. Blumgart L. H., Kelly C. J.: *Hepatojejunostomy in benign and malignant high bile duct strictures: approaches to the left hepatic ducts.* Br. J. Surg. 71: 257–61, 1984.
8. Bolondi L., Gaiani S., Testa S., Labò G.: *Gallbladder sludge formation during prolonged fasting after gastrointestinal tract surgery.* GUT 26: 734–738, 1985.

9. Chardavonne R., Kumari-Subhaya S., Auguste L. J., Philips G., Stein T. A., Wise L.: *Comparison of intraoperative ultrasonography and cholangiography in detection of small common bile duct stones.* Ann. Surg. 206: 52–55, 1987.

10. Chitwood W. R., Meyers W. C., Heaston D. K., Hrskovic A. M., Mc Leod M. E., Jones K. S.: *Diagnosis and treatment of primary extrahepatic bile duct tumor.* Am. J. Surg. 143: 99–106, 1982.

11. Custer M. D., Clore J. N.: *Source of error in operative cholangiography.* Arch. Surg. 100: 664–667, 1970.

12. De Gaetano A. M., Colagrande C., Boldrini G.: *L'ecografia intraoperatoria in chirurgia generale.* Us. Med. 3: 3–15, 1984.

13. Detich E. A.: *The reliability and clinical limitations of sonographic scanning of the biliary ducts.* Ann. Surg. 194: 167–170, 1981.

14. Dudely S. E., Edis A. J., Adson M. A.: *Biliary decompression in hilar obstruction. Round ligament approach.* Arch. Surg. 114: 519–522, 1972.

15. Eiseman B., Grenlaw R. H., Gallagher J. Q.: *Localization of common duct stones by ultrasound.* Arch. Surg. 91: 195–199, 1965.

16. Escalon A., Rosales W., Aldrete J.: *Reliability of pre- and intraoperative test for biliary lithiasis.* Ann. Surg. 201: 640–647, 1985.

17. Evander A., Fredlund P., Hovels H., Ihse I., Bengmark S.: *Evaluation of aggressive surgery for carcinoma of the extrahepatic bile ducts.* Ann. Surg. 191: 23–29, 1980.

18. Gazzaniga G. M., Faggioni A., Fialuro M.: *Surgical treatment of proximal bile duct tumors.* Int. Surg. 70: 45–48, 1985.

19. Gibby D. G., Hanks J. B., Wanebo H. J., Kaiser D. L., Tegtmeyer C. J., Chandler J. G., Jones R. S.: *Bile duct carcinoma. Diagnosis and treatment.* An.. Surg. 202: 139–145, 1985.

20. Gozzetti G., Principe A., Jovine E., Candeloro N., Cerretelli M.: *Il trattamento dei tumori dell'ilo epatico.* Chir. Epatobil. 4: 3–7, 1986.

21. Hall R. C., Sakiyalak P., Kim S. K. et al.: *Failure of operative cholangiography to prevent retained common duct stones.* Amm. J. Surg. 125: 51–57, 1973.

22. Hart M. J., White T. T.: *Central hepatic resection and anastomosis for structure or carcinoma at the hepatic bifurcation.* Ann. Surg. 192: 299–305, 1980.

23. Herbest C. A., Mittelstaedt C. A., Staab E. V., Buckwalter J. A.: *Intraoperative ultrasonography evaluation of the gallbladder in morbidly obese patients.* Ann. Surg. 200: 691–695, 1984.

24. Houssin D., Castaing D., Lemoine J. et al.: *Microlithiasis of the gallbladder.* Surgery Gynecol. Obstet. 157: 20–24, 1983.

25. Huguet C., Hakami F., Bloch P.: *L'intubation trans tumorale des obstructions néoplastiques du hile du foie. A propos de 36 observations.* Ann. Chir. 35: 341–347, 1981.

26. Jakimowicz J. J., Carol E. J., Jurgens P. T. H. J.: *The preoperative use of real time ultrasound imaging in biliary and pancreatic surgery.* Dig. Surg. 1: 55–60, 1984.

27. Jakimowicz J. J., Rutten H., Carol E., Jurgens P.: *Operative ultrasonography of the biliary tract.* Abstract 337, 1st World Congress Hepato-Pancreatico-Biliary Surgery, Lund, June 1986.

28. Knight R. P., Newell J. A.: *Operative use of ultrasonics in cholelitiasis.* Lancet 1: 1023–1025, 1963.

29. Lane R. J., Glazer G.: *Intraoperative B-mode ultrasound scanning of the intra-hepatic biliary system and pancreas.* Lancet 2: 334–337, 1980.

30. Lane R. J., Conpland G. A. E.: *Operative ultrasonic bile duct scanning.* Austr. N.Z.J. Surg. 49: 454–458, 1979.

31. Lane R. J., Craham A., Conpland G. A. E.: *Ultrasonic indications to explore the common bile duct.* Surgery 91: 268–274, 1982.

32. Langer I. C., Langer B., Taylor B. R., Zeldin R., Cummings B.: *Carcinoma of the extrahepatic bile ducts: results of an aggressive surgical approach.* Surgery 98: 752–759, 1985.

33. Launois B., Campion J. P., Brissot P., Gosselin M.: *Carcinoma of the hepatic hilus. Surgical management and the case for resection.* Ann. Surg. 190: 151–157, 1979.

34. Longmire W. P. Jr., Mc. Arthur M. S., Bastounis E. A., Hiatt J.: *Carcinoma of the extra-hepatic biliary tract*. Ann. Surg. 179: 345, 1973.
35. Machi J., Sigel B., Mc Crath E. C., Beitler J. C., Ramos J. R., Work B. A.: *Operative ultra-sonography in the biliary tract during pregnancy.* Surg. Gynecol. Obstet. 160: 119–123, 1985.
36. Ottow R., August D. A., Sugarbaker P. H.: *Treatment of proximal biliary tract carcinoma: an overview of techniques and results.* Surgery 97: 251–262, 1985.
37. Peracchia A., Baccaglini V., Tremolada C., Ferrarini M., Ruol A., Petri R., Castoro C., Da Vià G.: *Le protesi biliari in silastic.* Da: G. Gozzetti et al.. 'I tumori del fegato', Editrice Compositori, Bologna, pp. 254–259, 1985.
38. Plainfosse M. C., Merran S.: *Work in progress: intraoperative abdominal ultrasound.* Radiology 147: 829–832, 1983.
39. Plainfosse M. C., Alexandre J. H., Hernigou A. et al.: *Apport de l'echographie per-opéra-toire.* Presse Méd. 13: 1815–1817, 1984.
40. Puglionisi A., Nuzzo G., Magistrelli P., Costamagna G.: *Derivazioni intra-epatiche palliative nelle neoplasie dell'ilo epatico.* Chir. Epatobil. 1: 10–17, 1982.
41. Purdon R. C., Thomas S. R., Kerciakes J. G. et al.: *Ultrasonic properties of biliary calculi.* Radiology 136: 729–732, 1980.
42. Sigel B., Coelho J. C. U., Spigos D. G. et al.: *Real time ultrasonography during biliary surgery.* Radiology 137: 531–533, 1980.
43. Sigel B.: *Operative ultrasonography.* Lea and Fabinger Philadelphia, 1982.
44. Sigel B., Machi J., Beitler J. C. et al.: *Operative ultrasonography of pancreatic and biliary pathology.* Ann. Radiol. 25: 547–550, 1982.
45. Sigel B., Coelho J. C. U., Machi J., Flamangan D. P., Donahue P. E., Schuler J. J. N., Beitler J. C.: *The application of real time ultrasound imaging during surgical procedures.* Surg. Gynecol. Obstet. 157: 33–37, 1983.
46. Sigel B., Machi J., Beitherl J. C., Bonahue P. E., Bombeck T., Baker R. J., Duarte B.: *Comparative accuracy of operative ultrasonography and colangiography in detecting common duct calculi.* Surgery 94: 715–720, 1983.
47. Soupault R., Couninaud C.: *Sur un procédé nouveau de dérivation biliaire intrahépatique. Les cholangio-jejunostomies gauches sans sacrifice hépatique.* Presse Méd. 65: 1157–9, 1957.
48. Terblanche J., Saunders S., Louw J. H.: *Prolonged palliation in carcinoma of the main hepatic junction.* Surgery 71: 720–731, 1971.
49. Tremolada C., Baccaglini V., Ruol A., Ferrini M., Petri R., Castoro C., Lazzaro S., Pe-racchia A.: *Il ruolo dell'exeresi nel trattamento delle neoplasie primitive dell'ilo epatico.* Chir. Epatobil. 3: 21–24, 1984.
50. Tsuzuki T., Ogatr Y., Iida S. et al.: *Carcinoma of the bifurcation of the hepatic ducts.* Arch. Surg. 118: 1147–1151, 1983.
51. Vincent L. M., Mittlestaedt C. A.: *Intraoperative abdominal ultrasound.* In: Sauders R. C., Hillm., (Eds.): 'Ultrasound Annual 1984', Raven Press, New York, 1984.
52. Voyles C. R., Bowley N. Y., Allison D. J. et al.: *Carcinoma of the proximal extrahepatic biliary tree. Radiological assessment and therapeutic alternatives.* Ann. Surg. 197: 188–193, 1983.

Chapter 6: The role of intraoperative ultrasound in biliary surgery: results and critical evaluation in cholelithiasis and biliary cancer

J. F. GIGOT and P. J. KESTENS*

Introduction

The treatment of gallstone pathology (gallbladder lithiasis, common duct and intrahepatic stones) necessitates the detection of the stones and their complete removal from the bile ducts. Intraoperative ultrasound (IOUS) was introduced in biliary surgery in 1962 by Hayashi [27], Knight [33] and Eiseman [15], utilizing a mode-A ultrasound device whose pictures were difficult to analyze. Since the use of mode-B real-time ultrasound machines, different authors have shown the usefulness of IOUS as compared to intraoperative cholangiography for the detection of common duct stones [30, 31, 35–37, 50–56].

Although IOUS may be useful in biliary tumor surgery only a few publications [4] deal with this.

The aim of this study is to describe the technique of IOUS and to analyze the advantages and the limitations of this method in biliary stone and biliary tumor surgery.

Material and methods

Material

The IOUS machine is a linear real-time mode-B ultrasound (ALOKA-280)** using high frequency (5 and 7.5 mHz) sterile probes of different shapes. These probes are sterilized in a 2% glutaraldehyde solution for 20–30 minutes; there is no need to use a sterile bag since these probes are water tight. The surgeon himself manipulates the probes and is able to look at the echographic pictures on a video screen. Black and white photographs or a video recording can be taken from the screen. The machine can be adjusted by the operating room nurse and the presence of a radiologist or an X-ray technician is not required.

Methods

The IOUS is always performed before any surgical dissection and prior to the intraoperative cholangiogram. This avoids artefacts due to the presence of air

* Department of Surgery, University of Louven. Hôpital St. Luc, 10 Av. Hippocrate, Bruxelles.
** ALOKA BIOMEDIC – BELGIUM

98

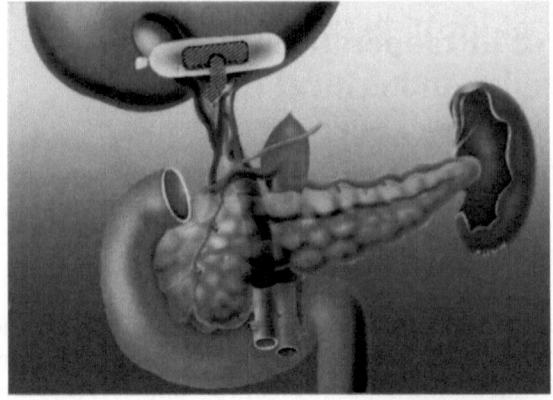

A

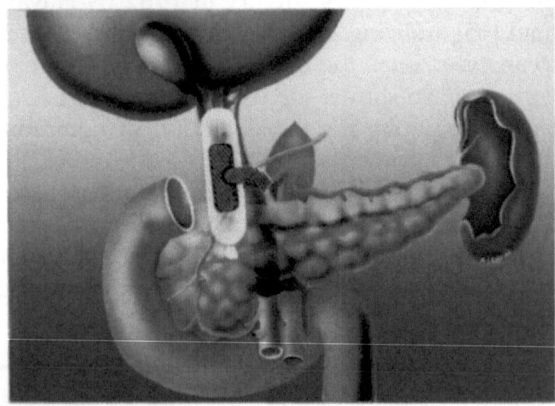

B

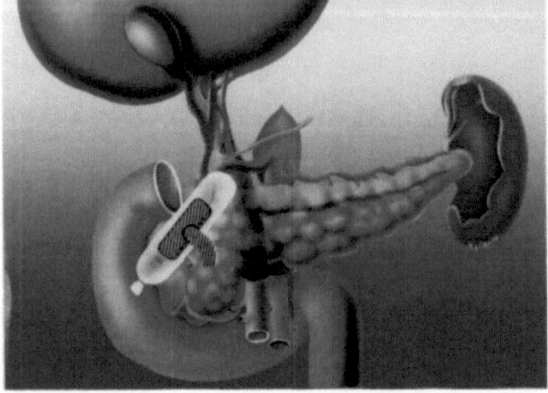

C

Figure 6.1. Different positions of the probe and the interposed water-filled balloon for intra-operative ultrasonic examination of the biliary system:

A) Application of the probe on the liver surface of segment IV: examination of the biliary convergence and the two main hepatic ducts.

B) Application of the probe on the anterior surface of the hepato-duodenal ligament: examination of the extra-pancreatic and extra-hepatic portion of the common bile duct.

C) Application of the probe on the anterior surface of the pancreatic head: examination of the intra-pancreatic portion of the common bile duct. The probe can be used with an interposed water-filled balloon on the posterior surface of the pancreatic head after Kocher manoeuvre.

in the tissues or tiny air bubbles trapped in the contrast medium injected into the biliary system.

The gallbladder, the main bile duct junction, the intrahepatic bile ducts are visualized by placing the probe directly on the surface of the liver. Trans-hepatic transverse and oblique scans are obtained by a 5 mHz (UST-587T-5) or a 7.5 mHz (UST-556T-7.5) flat T-shaped probe.

The gallbladder may be seen by placing the probe on the adjacent surfaces of segments IV and V, the main bile duct junction through the surface of segment IV (Fig. 6.1A) while the intrahepatic ducts are screened from the main junction up to the periphery of the liver by following the corresponding portal branches.

The extrahepatic supra-pancreatic common duct is visualized by transverse and sagittal scan through the liver parenchyma on the surface of segment IV and by caudally tilting the probe progressively over the surface of segment IV. However, the presence of air between the inferior aspect of segment IV and the anterior surface of the hepato-duodenal ligament may require the flood-ing of the area with saline used as a coupling agent as described by Sigel [54, 55].

One can also lift the inferior surface of segment IV and apply the probe to the surface of the hepato-duodenal ligament (Fig. 6.1B), either by immersion

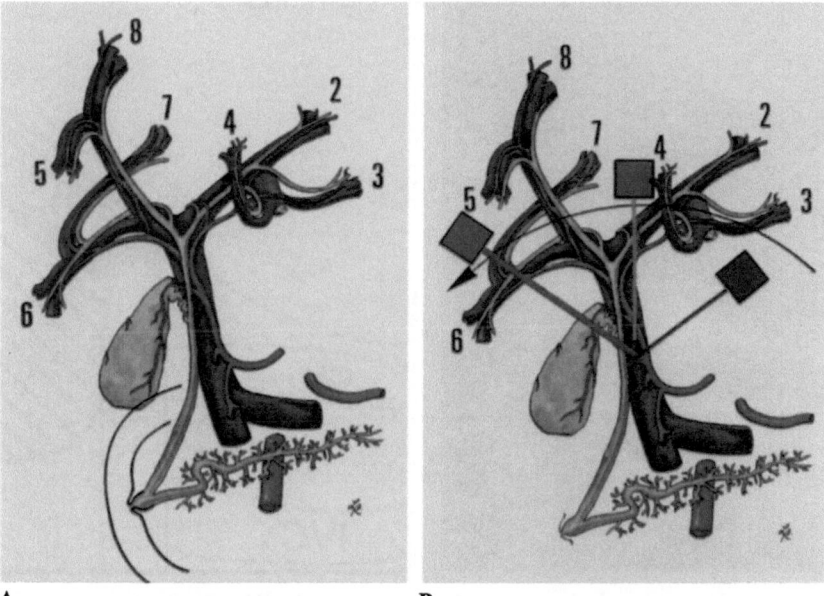

A   **B**

Figure 6.2. Positions of the probe for ultrasonic examination of the hepatoduodenal ligament:
A) Anatomy of the entire biliary tract.
B) Progressive axial rotation of the probe on the anterior surface of the hepato-duodenal liga-ment for sagittal scanning of the hepatic artery, the portal vein and the common bile duct.

of the area with saline or by interposing a water-filled balloon (i.e. a sterilized condom) [21, 22]. The vertical 7.5 mHz T-shaped probe (UST-556TU-7.5) is most appropriate for this purpose. Since the common duct is not exactly vertical but has a curved shape (oblique to the left with a concavity to the right), one has to modify the inclination of the probe on the surface of the hepato-duodenal ligament whose different components (hepatic artery, portal vein and common duct) are successively examined by gradually tilting the probe along its axis from left to right (Fig. 6.2).

The intra-pancreatic portion of the common duct is the most difficult to visualize down to the papilla of Vater. A Kocher manoeuvre can be helpful. The IOUS probe is placed either on the anterior surface of the duodenum and head of the pancreas (T-shaped probe of 7.5 mHz: UST-556TU-7.5 and UST–556T-7.5) (Fig. 6.1C) or at the posterior aspect of the duodeno-pancreatic block (T-shaped probe of 7.5 mHz: UST-556T-7.5) using a water-filled balloon as an interface between the probe and the above mentioned structures. The presence of air in the first part of the duodenum can jeopardize the quality of the echogram (Fig. 6.3). Therefore, one should evacuate the

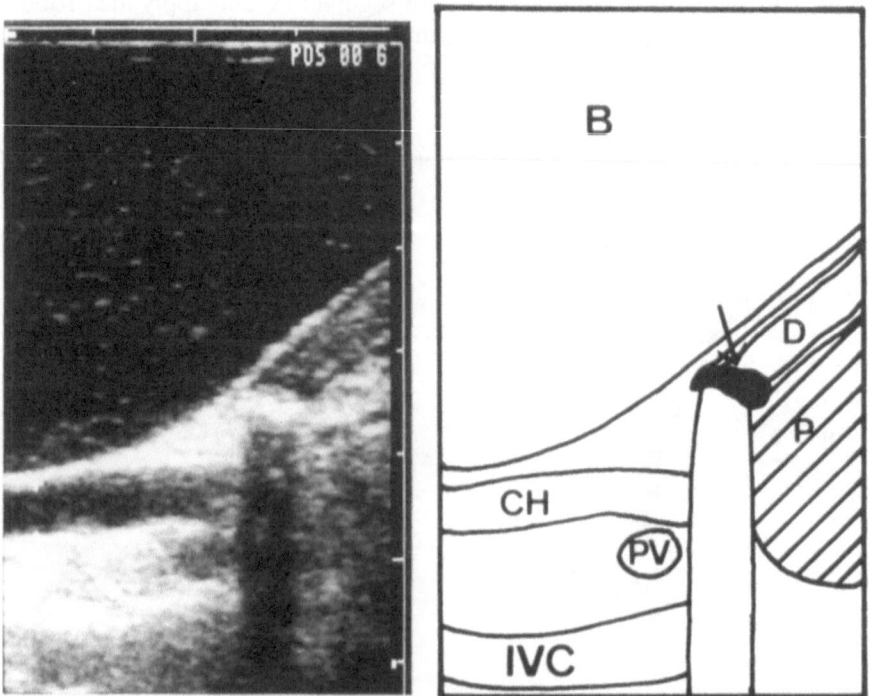

Figure 6.3. Sagittal scan at the lower part of the hepato-duodenal ligament: presence of gas (←) within the first part of the duodenum (D), giving artefacts for examination of the common bile duct (CH) at its entrance in the pancreatic head (P).
Posteriorly, oblique scan of the portal vein (PV) and sagittal scan of the inferior vena cava (IVC).

duodenum content by finger compression or by suction via a naso gastric tube introduced by the anaesthetist.

For the upper part of the common duct, gentle application of the probe without pressure is needed, in order to avoid collapse of the common duct lumen.

The ampulla of Vater is best seen by tracking the common duct downward first on sagittal scan, then on oblique scan as far as its junction with the Wirsung duct which becomes horizontal within the head of the pancreas.

By moving the probe from left to right during transverse scanning of the Wirsung duct at the posterior aspect of the head of the pancreas, it is also possible to examine the papilla. However, this procedure is difficult when the Wirsung duct is not dilated.

The IOUS can be performed through a subcostal or paramedian vertical incision. The mean duration of the IOUS depends on operator experience: at present, a complete diagnostic examination of the biliary tree takes an extra time of about 10 minutes.

The diameter of the bile ducts can be measured at any level by US scanning. Echoguided puncture of even a non dilated intra hepatic duct always allows an intraoperative cholangiogram. This selective puncture of the bile duct prevents the needle penetrating the portal branch with subsequent hemobilia. It is nevertheless mandatory to keep continuous echographic track of the tip of the needle when penetrating the bile duct, maintaining the needle strictly parallel to the ultrasound wave. The same principle is applied when performing echoguided biopsies for histologic examination of intrahepatic tumor masses.

Normal bile duct echoanatomy

The gallbladder appears as an anechogenic structure due to the bile contained in it, surrounded by a more echogenic area corresponding to the different layers of the gallbladder wall, measuring in normal conditions about 1–2 mm width. The cystic duct, in continuity with the gallbladder infundibulum, can sometimes be examined down to the junction with the common bile duct (Fig. 6.4) although its tortuosity often renders the echographic examination difficult (Fig. 6.5) if the biliary system is not dilated.

The intrahepatic bile ducts are located in front of the portal vein tree at the level of the glissonian pedicle, together with the corresponding branches of the portal vein and hepatic artery. When there is no dilatation, these bile ducts are hardly visible at the periphery of the liver parenchyma. On the contrary, they are always visualized at the level of the main bile duct junction (Fig. 6.6) appearing as tiny, thin walled, anechoic ducts parallel to the corresponding portal vein branch, the latter always being wider and surrounded by a more echogenic wall (Fig. 6.7). The arterial branch is recognized by its pulsatile nature during echoscopy. At the hilum, after locating the portal bifurcation,

102

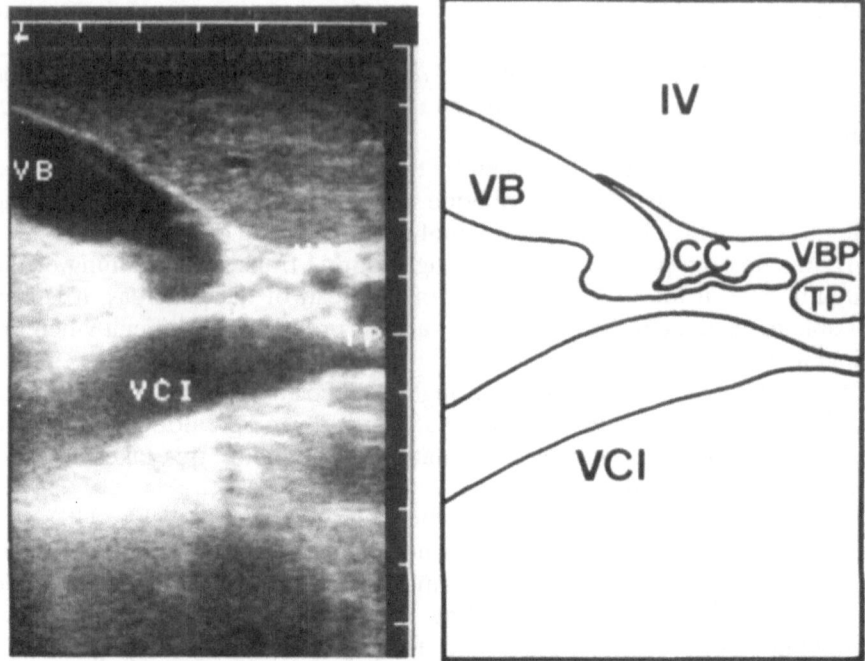

Figure 6.4. Transverse scan of the hepatic hilum: the cystic duct (CC) is very well visualized from the gallbladder (VB) to the common bile duct (VBP). Posteriorly, transverse scan of the portal vein (TP) and oblique scan of the inferior vena cava (VCI). Anteriorly, hepatic parenchyma of segment IV of Couinaud (IV).
With permission of Acta Gastro-Enterologica Belgica (18).

the main bile duct junction is examined by moving the probe slightly forward and upward.

The extrahepatic bile duct appears as an anechogenic thin-walled structure, measuring 4–5 mm in diameter under normal conditions and longitudinal on sagittal scan or more or less oval shaped on transverse. Between the hilum and the papilla, the axis of the common bile duct is modified: its direction is more or less vertical at the level of the common hepatic duct and then, slightly concave to the right, oblique downward and to the right, progressively joining the right side of the portal trunk. At this level, the right branch of the hepatic artery usually crosses the common hepatic duct. Further down, the common duct takes an oblique direction to the right, penetrating the upper part of the head of the pancreas, first having crossed the posterior aspect of the first part of the duodenum, while the portal trunk travels in an oblique direction down and to the left, posterior to the common duct. The direction of the hepatic artery within the hepato-duodenal ligament is even more oblique downward and to the left, becoming horizontal at the upper border of the head of the pancreas, after having given rise to the gastroduodenal artery which one can

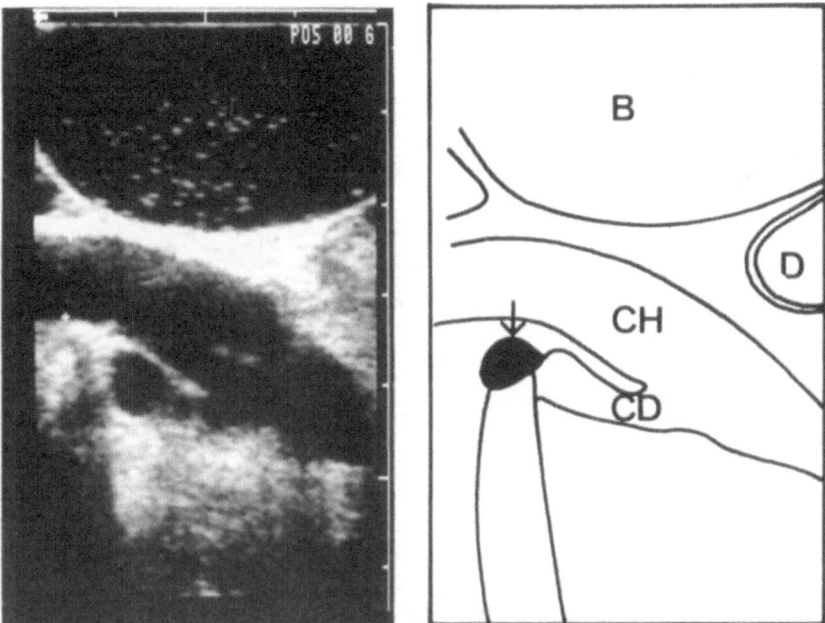

Figure 6.5. Sagittal scan of the hepatoduodenal ligament in a patient with dilatation of the extra-hepatic bile duct (CH). Posterior entrance of the cystic duct (CD) into the choledochus, with presence of a cystic duct stone (←). Interposed water-filled balloon (B). First part of the duodenum (D).

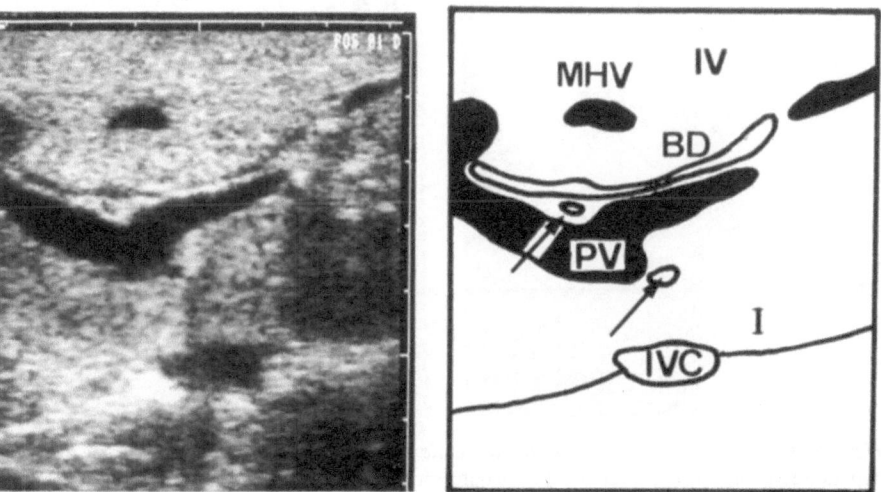

Figure 6.6. Transverse scan of the hepatic hilum. Presence of a normal biliary convergence (BD) above the portal convergence (PV). Division of the hepatic artery (←). Liver parenchyma of segment I and IV. Inferior vena cava (IVC).

104

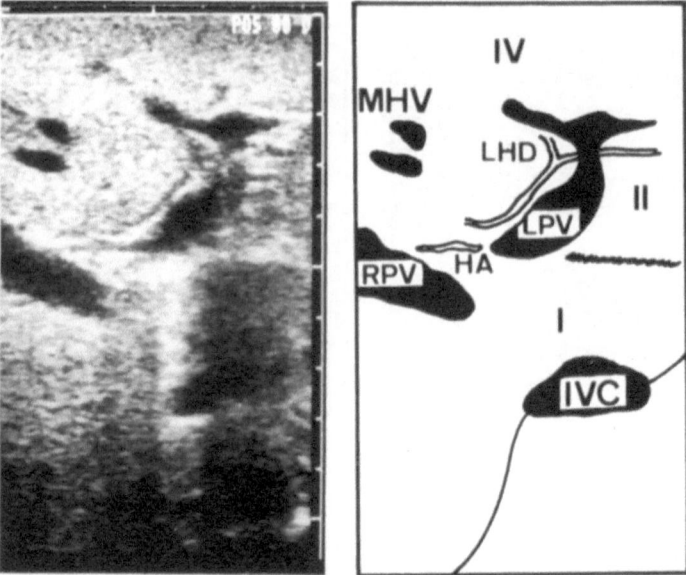

Figure 6.7. Transverse scan on the left side of the hepatic hilum: above and in front of the left portal vein (LPV), presence of a normal left hepatic duct (LHD). Left branch of the hepatic artery (HA). Right portal vein (RPV). Middle hepatic vein (MHV). Inferior vena cava (IVC). Hepatic parenchyma of segment I, II and IV.

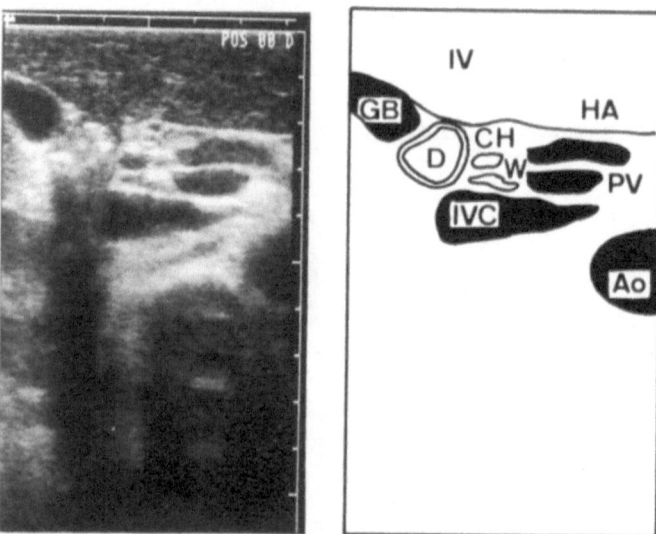

Figure 6.8. Transverse scan of the intrapancreatic portion of the common bile duct using trans-hepatic scanning through segment IV: visualization of the distal part of the choledochus (CH) and the Wirsung duct (W) in the pancreatic head. On the right side of the choledochus, presence of the duodenum (D) and the neck of the gallbladder (GB). On the left side, presence of the hepatic artery (HA) and the portal vein (PV). Posteriorly, inferior vena cava (IVC) and aorta (AO).

easily follow on sagittal scanning between the superior aspect of the head of the pancreas and the posterior wall of the first part of the duodenum. These three structures (hepatic artery, portal vein and common duct) are thus examined successively on sagittal scan by gradually tilting the ultrasound probe on its axis from left to right (Fig. 6.2).

In its intrapancreatic portion, the extra hepatic bile duct becomes even more oblique to the right where it joins the papilla at the level of the second part of the duodenum. On transverse scan (Fig. 6.8), the common bile duct is located to the right of the intrapancreatic portion of the superior mesenteric vein and approaches the internal border of the second part of the duodenum (Fig. 6.9). The papilla appears as an outgrowth of the duodenal mucosa at the junction of the common bile and Wirsung ducts (Fig. 6.10). In normal conditions, the latter can be distinguished within the head of the pancreas as two parallel thin echogenic lines measuring 1–2 mm in diameter.

Thus, IOUS may be of value in localizing the bile ducts in case of acute cholecystitis, inflammatory process of the hepato-duodenal ligament or in further biliary surgery, thereby avoiding operative trauma of the main bile duct during a difficult surgical resection.

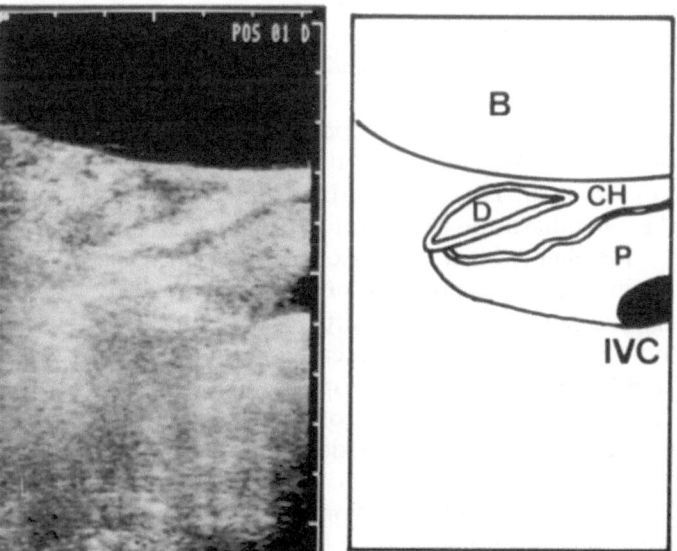

Figure 6.9. Oblique scan of the pancreatic head (P). Excellent visualization of the choledochus (CH) down to its entrance into the second part of the duodenum (D). Inferior vena cava (IVC).

106

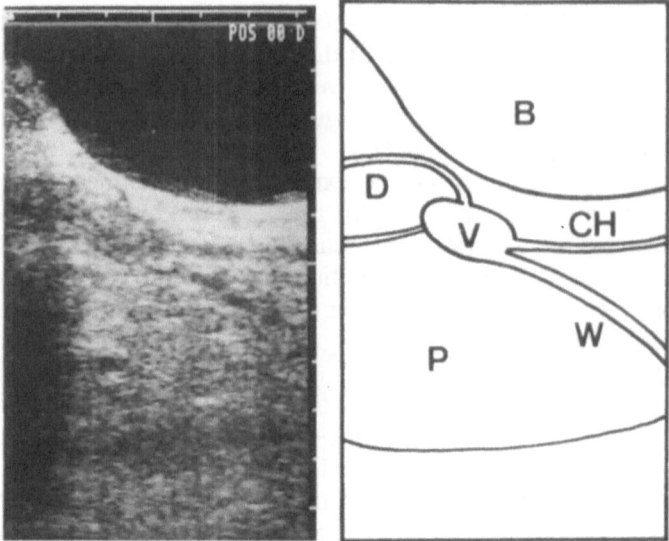

Figure 6.10. Scanning of the intra-pancreatic portion of the common bile duct, with an interposed water-filled balloon (B) behind the head of the pancreas (P). Excellent visualization of the intra-pancreatic choledochus (CH) and the Wirsung duct (W) and their confluence at the level of the ampulla of Vater (V), in the second part of the duodenum (D).

Lithiasis

1. Gallbladder

The echographic semiology of gallbladder lithiasis is classical: a hyperechogenic picture with a posterior acoustic shadow. The sensitivity of preoperative ultrasound in the detection of gallstones measuring more than 5 mm in diameter is close to 100%. The use of IOUS for the diagnosis of gallbladder lithiasis is thus minimal. However, Herbst [28] has shown that IOUS detected 16% of unknown lithiasis on preoperative examination and after peroperative palpation – together with 1.8% false positives corresponding to parietal granuloma – in 55 patients operated on for morbid obesity. The palpation of stones within the gallbladder is also difficult when there is a thick-walled gallbladder (cholecystitis, cirrhosis) or in case for an intrahepatic gallbladder [4]. When there is no preoperative work-up (in an emergency case for example) or during a non biliary operation (colon surgery, cirrhosis...), IOUS may prove useful in the detection of gallbladder stones [4].

On the other hand, the diagnosis of microlithiasis is often missed by preoperative ultrasound and palpation, even in a patient with a previous history of relapsing acute pancreatitis [4]. As well as others, we have seen a few patients with microlithiasis in whom no stones were found on preoperative ultrasonography (Fig. 6.11).

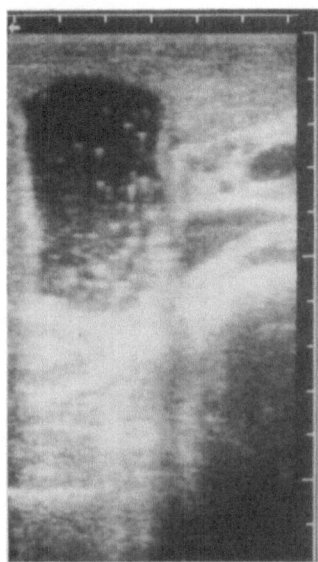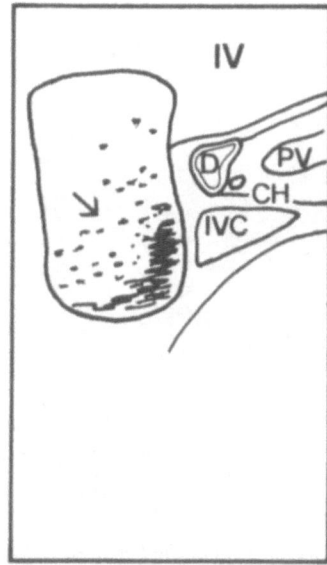

Figure 6.11. Normal preoperative ultrasound and intraoperative palpation of the gallbladder in this patient operated upon for chronic pancreatitis.
On this *traverse scan of the hepatic hilum*, presence of multiple microlithiasis in the gallbladder. Transverse scan of the portal vein (PV), the common bile duct (CH), the inferior vena cava (IVC) and the duodenum (D).

The diagnosis of microlithiasis is based on the detection of small sized intraluminal echoes, appearing as deposits within the lumen of the gallbladder; the ultrasonic waves being partially absorbed after having passed through the sediment. Indeed, a real acoustic shadow is not only visible in these cases of microlithiasis but also when cholesterolic stones or sludge are present [37]. The 'sludge' or 'hyperechogenic bile' corresponds to an echogenic intraluminal content which is relatively homogeneous, without deposits in the gallbladder lumen and without posterior absorption of the echoes. This echographic picture of the sludge is probably due to modifications of the lipidic composition of the gallbladder bile. An echogenic picture without posterior acoustic shadow, fixed in the gallbladder lumen and especially if attached to the gallbladder wall, corresponds to a polyp or parietal granuloma. Parietal inflammatory changes (acute cholecystitis) or tumors (gallbladder cancer) can also be easily detected.

2. Common duct stones

Many authors have shown that 15–25% of the patients operated on for biliary stones had an exploratory choledoctomy [13, 14, 32, 58]. The incidence of residual stones after choledocotomy varies in the literature from 1 to 10% with a mean of 4% [14, 24, 46, 58]. Nevertheless, the systematic and strict use

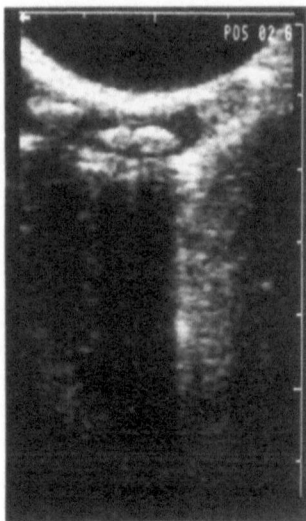 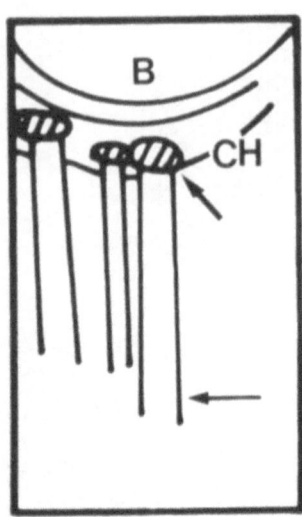

Figure 6.12. Sagittal scan of the hepato-duodenal ligament using an interposed water-filled balloon (B): presence of three stones in the common bile duct (CH): hyperechogenic image (←) with an acoustic shadow (←).

of peroperative cholangioscopy and -graphy and of the choledoscope by experienced teams can lower this incidence to about 2% [3, 16].

The echographic criteria of stones in the common bile duct (Figs. 6.12, 6.13) are well defined: a hyperechogenic picture (sensitivity 88%, specificity 94%) which persists on decreasing the attenuation of the US beam, with a posterior acoustic shadow (sensitivity 84%, specificity 95%); in most cases there is dilatation of the upper common bile duct, the diameter of which is superior or equal to 10 mm (sensitivity 72%, specificity 92%) [36, 37]. The sensitivity of preoperative ultrasonography in the diagnosis of common duct stones is 40% in Kunstlinger's experience [17] with a specificity of 90% and a positive predictive value of 80%. Quite a few articles [30, 31, 37, 54, 55, 56] have compared the value of echography and peroperative cholangiogram in the detection of common bile duct stones: IOUS is superior to cholangiogram in terms of efficiency [31] and positive predictive value [55, 56]. Two experimental studies – in vivo [8] and in vitro [40] – have also demonstrated that echography is superior to cholangiogram in the detection of small stones down to a diameter of 1 mm [40] (Fig. 6.14). The sensitivity of cholangiography for small sized stones is indeed linked to the size of the common bile duct and to the concentration of the contrast medium [40]. Nevertheless, it seems difficult to extrapolate the results of these series in our practice without taking into account a few elements: firstly the number of negative choledocotomies performed in these series is relatively high: 12% [55, 56]; 19% [37]; 24% [31] and 29% [30]. In addition, an intraoperative cholangiogram is omitted in many cases (19% for Sigel) [55] or fails or is impossible to achieve

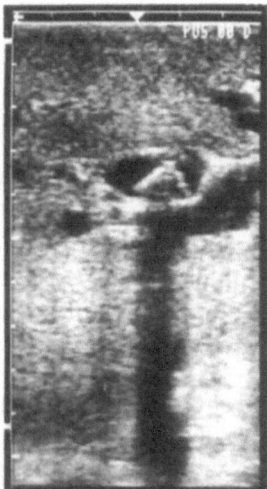 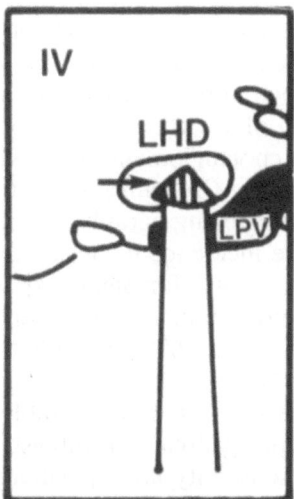

Figure 6.13. Transverse scan of the left part of the hepatic hilum: presence of a stone (→) in the dilated left hepatic duct (LHD) above the left portal vein (LPV). Hepatic parenchyma of segment IV of Couinaud (IV).

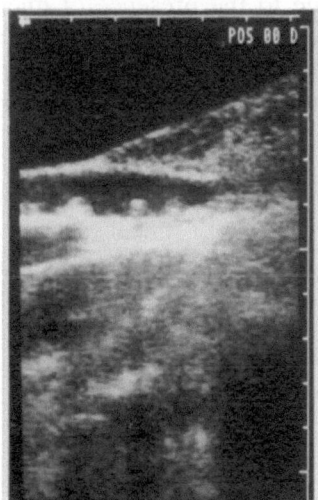 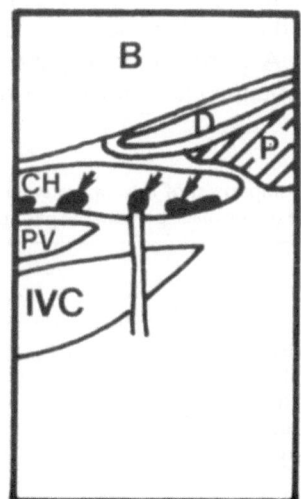

Figure 6.14. Sagittal scan of the common bile duct (CH) at the lower part of the hepato-duodenal ligament, with a interposed water-filled balloon (B): on the right, first part of the duodenum (D) and pancreatic head (P). Presence of multiple microlithiasis (←) in the choledochus (CH).
Posteriorly, presence of the portal vein (PV) and the inferior vena cava (IVC).

for technical reasons: 5% for Jakimowicz [31], 12% for Lane [37], or else cannot be interpreted or is not technically satisfactory: 5% for Lane [37], 5% for Sigel [55], 4% for Jakimowicz [30]. Moreover, the peroperative cholangiography described in these articles usually involves 3 successive X-ray pictures after injection of a certain amount of contrast medium, without fluoroscopy or associated cholangiomanometry which is generally the rule in France [3, 4] or in our country (Belgium). Nevertheless, systematic use of IOUS in conjunction with cholangiography is highly beneficial (23% for Lane) [37], decreasing the incidence of negative choledocotomy: 21 to 7% for Jakimowicz [30]; 19 to 14% for Sigel [54]. The combination of peroperative ultrasonography and cholangiography permits the detection of unrecognized common duct stones in 3.6% [30] to 7% [31] of patients, and residual stones in less than 1% [31].

In our personal experience (Table 1) [23], of a prospective series of 70 patients (simple gallbladder lithiasis: [37]; gallbladder and common duct stones: [33], sensitivity and specificity is 93.9% and 97.3% respectively for echography; and 92.6% and 94.6% for intraoperative cholangiography. Predictive value for echography is 96.9% and 92.6% for cholangiography. Combined use of both methods was able, in this series, to avoid any negative choledocotomy and residual common duct stones. Regarding the total number of stones, intraoperative cholangiogram detected 79.6% of them, IOUS 94% and the combination of IOUS + cholangiogram, 100% of common duct stones. False positives for cholangiography (2/37) and IOUS (1/37) are due to air bubbles in the bile ducts. False negatives during peroperative cholangiography (2/27) are due to the presence of micro calculi just above the papilla which is a particularly difficult area to explore using this technique. A retro-duodeno-pancreatic approach for IOUS of the common bile duct obtained after a Kocher manoeuvre facilitates the ultrasonic exami-

Table 6.1. Comparison of intraoperative ultrasonography and cholangiography in detection of common bile duct stones: personal experience

	Ultrasonography (n = 70)	Cholangiography (n = 64)
– True positive :	31/33	25/27
– True negative :	36/37	35/37
– False positive :	1/37	2/37
– False negative :	2/33	2/27
– Technically unsatisfactory :	1	1
– Sensitivity (%) :	93.9	92.6
– Specificity (%) :	97.3	94.6
– Accuracy (%) :	95.7	93.8
– Predictive value of a negative test (%) :	94.7	94.6
– Predictive value of a positive test (%) :	96.9	92.6
– Prevalence of CBD stones (%) :	47.1	42.2

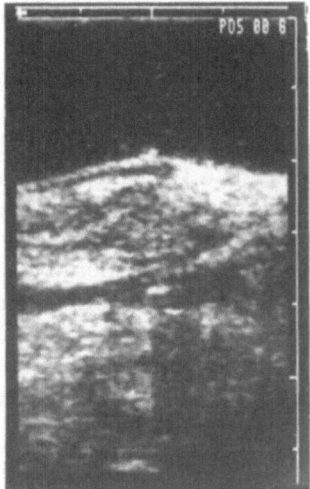 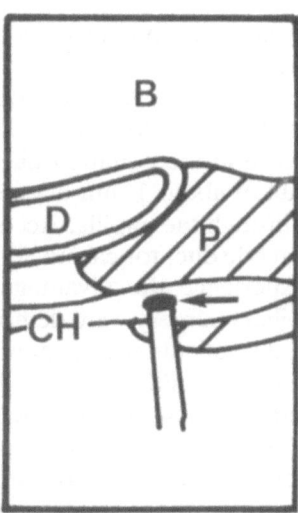

Figure 6.15. Sagittal scan of the lower part of the hepato-duodenal ligament, using a interposed water-filled balloon (B): presence of a small stone (←) in the pancreatic portion of the chole-dochus (CH). Pancreatic head (P) and first portion of the duodenum (D).

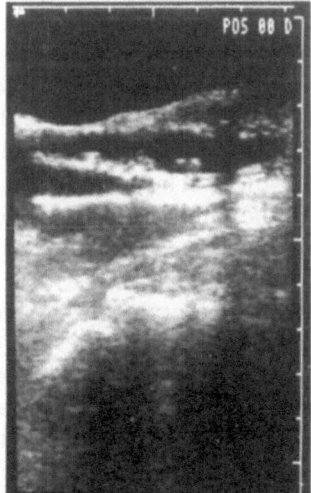 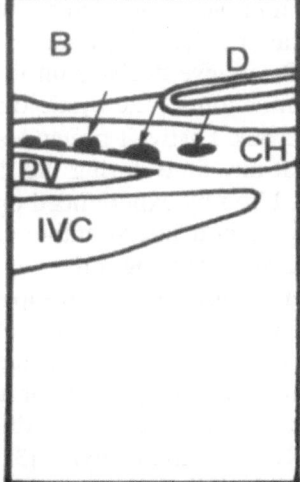

Figure 6.16. Transverse scan of the hepato-duodenal ligament, with and interposed water-filled balloon (B). Presence of *microlithiasis and gravel* (←) in the choledochus (CH). First part of the duodenum (D). Posteriorly to the common bile duct, presence of the portal vein (PV) and the inferior vena cava (IVC).

nation and the detection of stones in the lower intra-pancreatic common bile duct [8] (Fig. 6.15).

However, strict echographic criteria should be adhered to in opting for an exploratory choledocotomy because, due to its high resolution power, IOUS can detect within the common bile duct lumen, the presence of sludge and micro calculi of about 1 mm diameter [40] (Fig. 6.16) which may pass spontaneously through the papilla. According to Lane [37], one should only open the common bile duct for calculi about 3 mm in diameter or greater.

In our experience, the advantages of IOUS over intraoperative cholangiography in biliary surgery were demonstrated in 11.4% of all our patients n=70) and among 33 patients with common duct stones (8 patients: 24.2%): 2 with an overlooked microlithiasis at cholangiography, 4 with a better estimation of the total number of stones; in one patient, a diagnosis of benign lesion was confirmed on histology of a suspect nodule in the head of the pancreas and finally a stone impacted in the common bile duct was diagnosed in a patient operated on for suspected bile duct cancer (Fig. 6.17).

Compared to the intraoperative cholangiogram, the advantages of IOUS are multiple [30, 31, 37, 54, 55, 56]: it is a non invasive technique, involving no x-rays or contrast medium. These characteristics are most beneficial when biliary surgery has to be performed on a pregnant woman. In which case, IOUS can replace the peroperative cholangiogram, as described by Machi [41]. We have, in our experience, operated upon 2 such patients suffering from biliary acute pancreatitis. When it is impossible to introduce a canula to the cystic duct, IOUS can replace the intraoperative X-ray. No contra-indication to ultrasound is known and it can be achieved more rapidly than intraoperative cholangiogram. IOUS is cheaper, repeatible and instantaneous, delivering multiple plane pictures. Its resolution capacity is about 1 mm and one can examine the liver, pancreas and surrounding structures at the same time. IOUS can give decisive information before any surgical dissection and without canulation of the cystic duct which can sometimes be difficult and even dangerous. Lastly, it precludes the presence of a radiologist during the operation at any time during the day or at night. The technique constantly progresses. Used by experienced operators the number of failures or of non satisfactory or non interpretable examinations appears to be less than for intraoperative cholangiogram.

However, compared to intraoperative cholangiogram, IOUS has certain disadvantages [30, 31, 37, 54, 55, 56]: IOUS does not permit complete visualization of the bile duct anatomy as does intraoperative cholangiogram and does not show the passage of fluid through the papilla. The examination of the intrapancreatic common duct, especially close to the papilla necessitates a Kocher manoeuvre [31, 54, 55], a retro-duodeno-pancreatic approach to the bile duct [52] or flooding the surgical field with sterile saline [31, 53, 54, 55].

Several adapted probes are needed to detect the different location of the stones: flat 5 mHz T-shaped probes for intrahepatic lithiasis, vertical 7.5 mHz

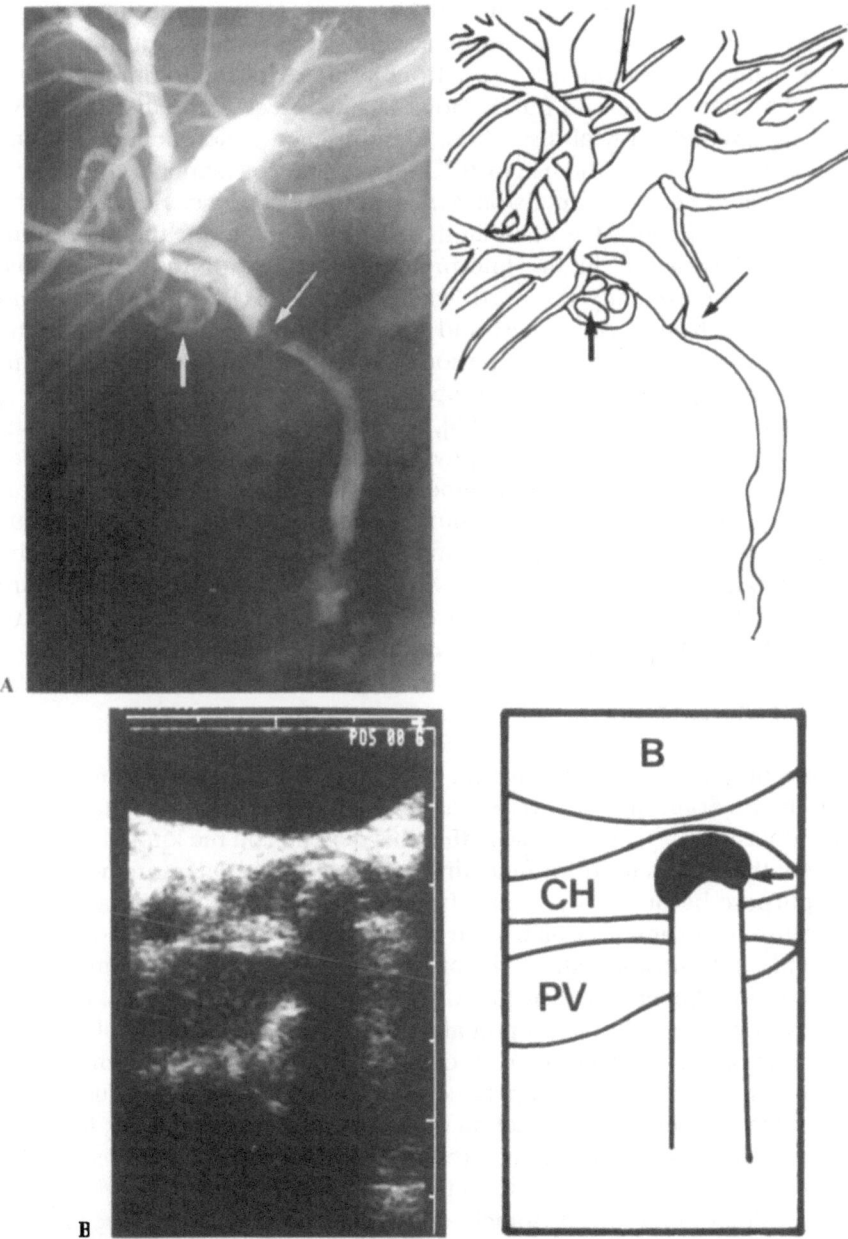

Figure 6.17.
A) *Trans-hepatic cholangiogram:* presence of *multiple gallstones* (←), with a stenosis in the middle part of the common bile duct (←) presenting an irregular aspect and a convex upper border, which is suspected to be a tumoral lesion.

B) *Sagittal scan of the hepato-duodenal* ligament with an interposed water-filled balloon (B) in the same patient. At the level of the radiological stenosis, ultrasound demonstrates a *typical picture of stone*, with hyperechogenic image (←) and acoustic shadow. Posteriorly to the choledochus (CH), presence of the portal vein (PV).

T-shaped probes for the hepato-duodenal ligament. The presence of air in the duodenum and the existence of aerobilia (endoscopic sphincterotomy, biliary digestive fistula or anastomoses...) are troublesome for echographic examination [37, 55]. For this reason IOUS should always precede the intraoperative cholangiogram and surgical dissection. The presence of aerobilia after stone extraction thus prevents the use of IOUS as a control examination for complete removal of common duct stones: this, in our experience, is achieved by choledocoscopy. Finally, the main limitation of the method is the general inexperience of surgeons in the interpretation and use of the echographic pictures and consequently the need, when starting IOUS, for technical and diagnostic help from a radiologist and intensive training before the routine use of this method. However, this period of training is longer for IOUS compared with intraoperative cholangiography.

In contrast to others [30, 31, 37, 55], we believe that IOUS is not a substitute for intraoperative cholangiography but rather that these two techniques are complementary. Sigel [56] recommends IOUS as the unique intraoperative technique in the detection of common bile duct stones in an anicterous patient and when the size of the common duct is normal. He advocates the use of IOUS as a first step in patients with jaundice and when bile ducts are dilated: this also avoids intraoperative cholangiography if IOUS is positive and if one does not suspect disease of the sphincter of Oddi.

3. Intrahepatic stones

There are only a few publications [2, 3, 25] on the use of IOUS for intrahepatic stones. Some authors [31, 37] assume that it is difficult to detect intrahepatic lithiasis by IOUS: we believe that this depends on the kind of material employed; the probes used for detecting common duct stones, are not suited to this purpose because they cannot be fitted underneath the costal margin and because they cannot visualize the entire liver parenchyma. Preoperative ultrasound and intraoperative cholangiography often underestimate the presence of intrahepatic lithiasis [3, 26, 34]. For intrahepatic stones, IOUS is used only in patients operated upon after the failure of non surgical therapy (endoscopic or transhepatic removal of stones, extracorporeal or endoluminal lithotripsy...) or in patients operated on for complicated and diffuse intrahepatic lithiasis when a liver resection might be necessary [1, 10, 44, 49]. The diagnostic criteria for assuming the presence of intrahepatic stones have to be strict: intraluminal hyperechogenic pictures with acoustic shadows – as in any lithiasis – alongside a portal branch and usually associated with segmental dilatation of the intrahepatic bile duct. The intrahepatic stones must thus be distinguished from aerobilia (hyperechogenic signals with a posterior acoustic shadow equivalent to a lithiasis but thinner and more variable in positions and features), from granulomas or hepatic parenchymal calcifications (located outside the portal branch areas in the middle of the hepatic parenchyma), or from a transverse scan of the peripheral venous, arterial and biliary elements (corrected by moving the probe in multiple planes). In our experience, 5 patients had an intrahepatic lithiasis: five patients had multiple stones and 3 patients had one, occupying one lobe in 6 patients and 2 lobes in 2.

The value of IOUS is threefold:

1. detection of intrahepatic stones;
2. their precise topographic localization within the hepatic parenchyma;
3. the detection of an associated intrahepatic abscess due to cholangitis (Figs. 6.18, 6.19, 6.20).

IOUS can be helpful in performing an intraperative cholangiogram via echoguided puncture of the obstructed segmental hepatic duct which, of course, cannot be visualized by a standard intraoperative cholangiogram [2].

From a therapeutic point of view, the use of IOUS can limit the extent of the hepatic resection – whenever indicated – to the one segment or sector of the liver containing the stones [4, 23, 25]. It also permits echoguided removal of the stones during the operation as well as intubation of the intrahepatic bile ducts for postoperative percutaneous access, intrahepatic dilatation of associated bile duct stenoses [4] as well as guided hepatotomies for removal of intrahepatic lithiasis [9, 43].

Persistence of residual intrahepatic stones detected by IOUS lead in our experience to hepatectomy in some patients and in others, to the implantation of a U-shaped Praderi type transhepatic drainage device for postoperative removal of stones by external manoeuvre. Theoretically, an intraluminal lithotrypsy (by electrohydraulic or ultrasonic probe) can be performed during

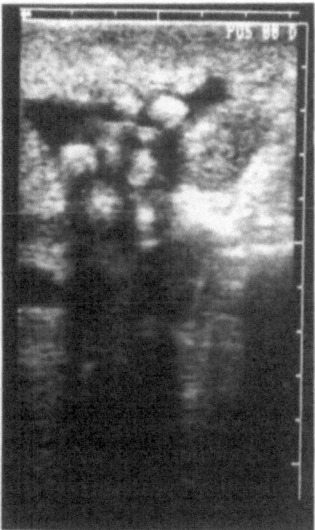 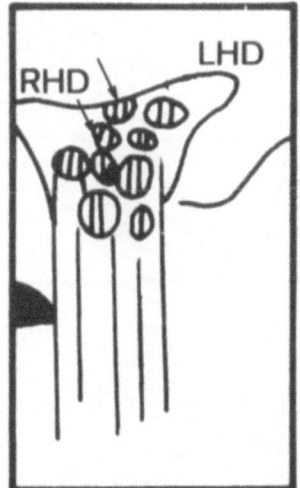

Figure 6.18. Transverse scan of the hepatic hilum: presence of *multiple stones* (←) at the junction between the right hepatic duct (RHD) and the left hepatic duct (LHD).

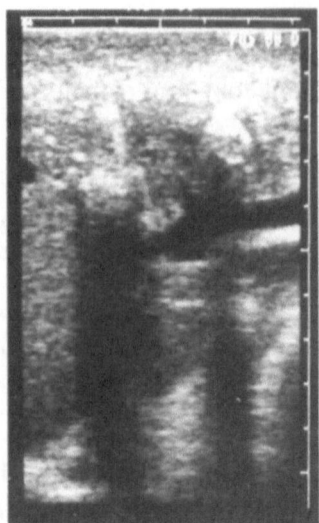 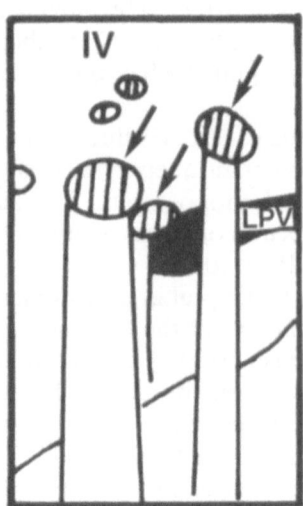

Figure 6.19. Transverse scan of the left part of the hepatic hilum: Multiple intra-hepatic stones (←) occupying completely the left hepatic duct which is no longer visible, above the left portal vein (LPV). Hepatic parenchyma of segment IV (IV) of Couinaud.

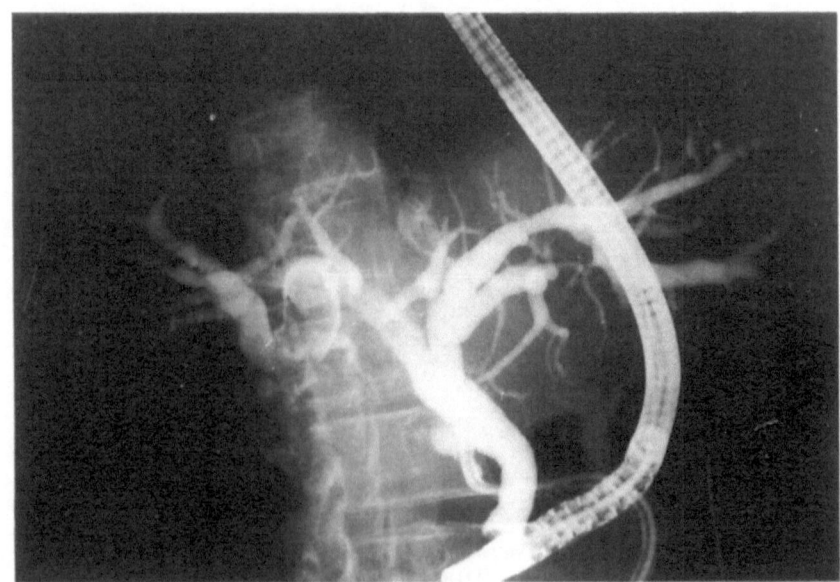

A

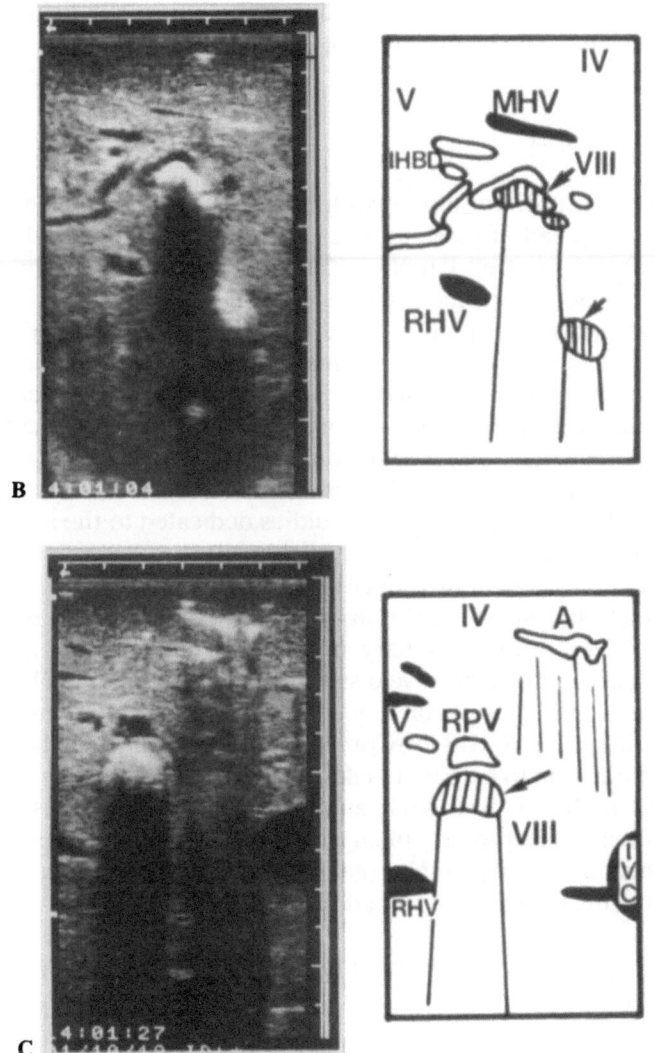

Figure 6.20. Patient with right intrahepatic stones.
A) Preoperative ERCP.
B) Transverse scan of the hepatic hilum: segment IV of Couinaud (IV) above the middle hepatic vein (MHV). In the antero-medial sector (segment V and VIII) of the right liver – between the middle hepatic vein (MHV) and the right hepatic vein (MHV) – presence of an intra-hepatic stone, with an hyperechogenic image (←) with an acoustic shadow, associated to dilatation of an intra-hepatic bile duct (IHBD). In the postero-lateral sector of the right liver (segment VI and VII), behind the right hepatic vein (RHV), presence of another intra-hepatic stone (←).
C) Transverse scan of the hepatic hilum in the same patient: inferior vena cava (IVC). Presence of aerobilia (A) in segment IV of Couinaud (IV). In the right antero-medial sector of the liver, presence of an obstructive intra-hepatic stone (←) in the right hepatic duct, close to the right portal vein (RPV).

combined endoscopy and echoscopy through a loop of the jejunum, anastomosed at the hilum and externally accessible via a stoma.

Tumors of the bile duct

The diagnostic approach for tumors of the bile ducts consists mainly in determining the local spread of these tumors [11, 19, 45, 57, 59]: the discovery of hepatic metastases, invaded lymph nodes and vascular involvement are the limiting factors when choosing – before or during the operation – treatment of a particular patient, keeping in mind the difficulties of resective surgery. Long postoperative survival, with optimal quality of life [39] and low postoperative mortality and morbidity justify aggressive wide resection of the lesions including associated resection of segment I [29, 42], vascular reconstruction after removal of vein segments [7, 48], or total hepatectomy and transplantation [47]. The resectability rate of these cancers varies between 10 and 30% [5, 6, 18, 20, 38]. Only a few studies dedicated to the advantages of using IOUS in this type of surgery are available [4].

Usually, the preoperative investigations (ultrasound, CT-scan, cholangiography, arteriography) in patients with obstructive jaundice try to determine the nature of the underlying biliary obstruction and regional spread of a tumor. During operation, extensive dissection of the hilum of the liver is often necessary to evaluate the resectability of these tumors. Before embarking on any surgical dissection IOUS can provide the surgeon with the necessary diagnostic information to help him make this decision.

The *results of IOUS* have been analyzed in a prospective series of 27 patients with malignant primary biliary obstruction (hilum: 16, common bile duct: 4) or secondary malignancies (gallbladder cancer: 6 and hepatic tumor extending up to the main hepatic junction: 1).

1. Detection, topographic localization and biliary extension of the tumors of the bile ducts

At the hilum, the tumor appears as a hypo or iso-echogenic mass, heterogeneous, with ill-defined contours – due to the infiltrative characteristics of the tumor – interrupting the main bile duct junction (Fig. 6.21).

The extension of the tumor distally to the junction of the secondary biliary bifurcations (Fig. 6.22) and proximally to the common bile duct – easily examined by IOUS – constitute important data when deciding what surgical technique should be used. Endoprosthesis or transtumoral tubes when present for a long period of time, complicate the evaluation of this parietal extension because of a mural inflammatory process of the bile ducts due to the presence of a foreign body.

At the level of the extra (Fig. 6.23) and intra-pancreatic common bile duct (Fig. 6.24), the bile duct tumor appears as a hypoechogenic mass in com-

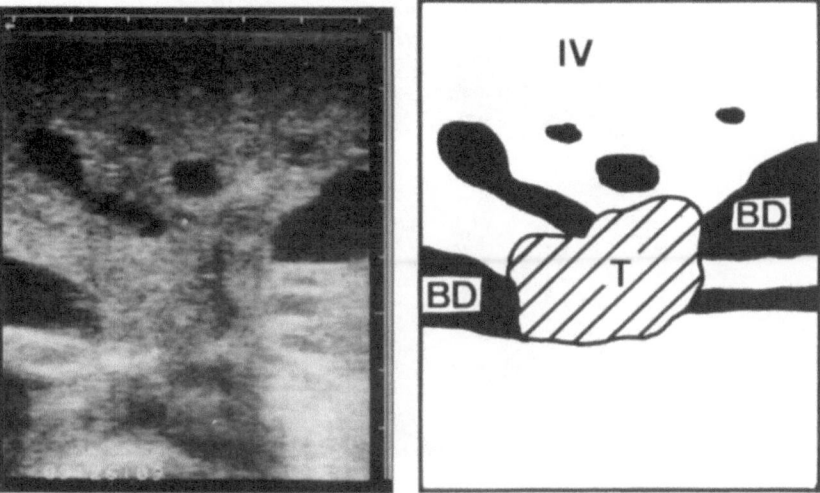

Figure 6.21. Transverse scan of the hepatic hilum: interruption of the intra-hepatic bile duct (BD) by an *hypoechogenic hilar tumor* (T).
With permission of Acta Gastro-Enterologica Belgica (18).

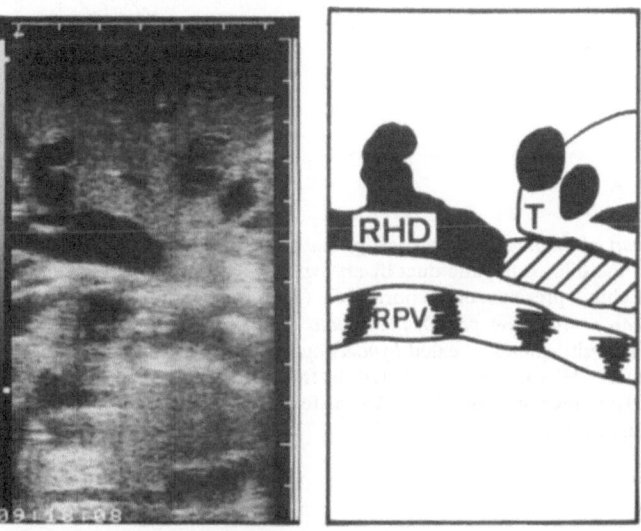

Figure 6.22. Transverse scan of the right side of the hepatic hilum in the same patient: *invasion of the right hepatic duct* (RHD) by the hilar tumor (T). Posteriorly, right portal vein (RPV). With permission of Acta-Gastro-Enterologica Belgica (18).

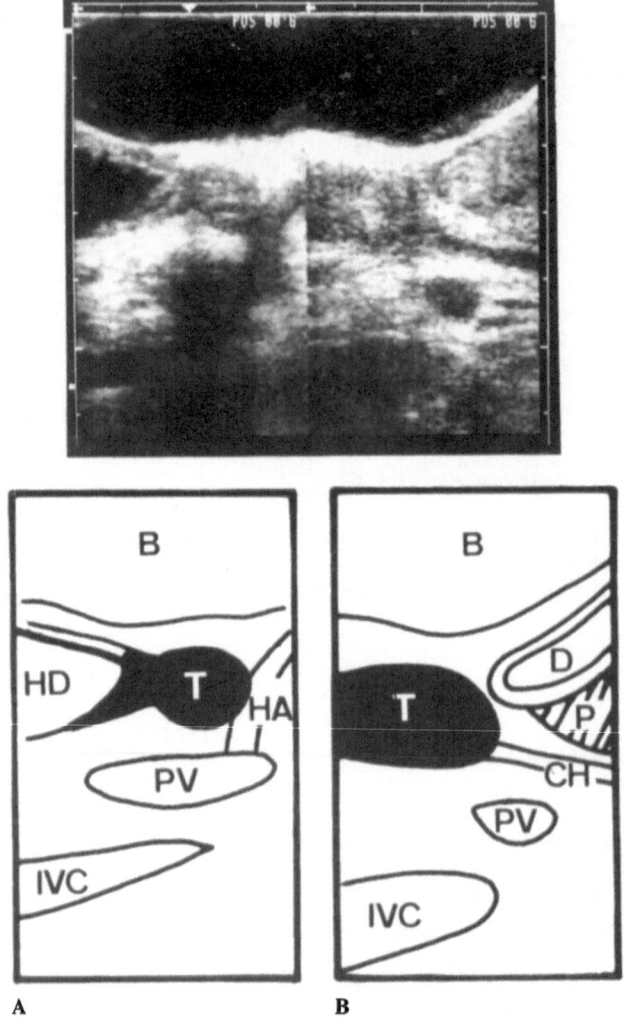

Figure 6.23.

A) *Sagittal scan of the hepato-duodenal ligament* with an interposed water filled balloon (B): obstruction of the dilated hepatic duct by an *hypoechogenic tumor* (T): invasion of the hepatic artery (HA). Behind, presence of the portal vein (PV) and the inferior vena cava (IVC).

B) *Sagittal scan at the lower part of the hepato duodenal ligament* with an interposed water-filled balloon (B): ultrasound revealed *hypoechogenic tumor* (T) and the intra-pancreatic part of the choledochus (CH) which is not dilated. In front of the common bile duct, first part of the duodenum (D) and the pancreatic head (P). Posteriorly, oblique scan of the portal vein (PV) and the inferior vena cava (IVC).

parison with the surrounding structures of the hepato-duodenal ligament, lying in the area of the common duct and interrupting its lumen. In the obstructive jaundiced patient operated upon for a suspected tumor of the bilio-pancreatic area, IOUS has indicated on several occasions the difference between a primary cholangiocarcinoma (irregular thickening of the bile duct wall centered by the common duct tumor) (Fig. 6.24) or a primary adeno-carcinoma of the pancreas (intrapancreatic tumoral mass, invading the common duct with a mass extending eccentrically to the lumen of the common bile duct) (Figs. 6.25–6.26). The diagnosis of tumor of the ampulla of Vater is also possible by IOUS (Fig. 6.27).

A

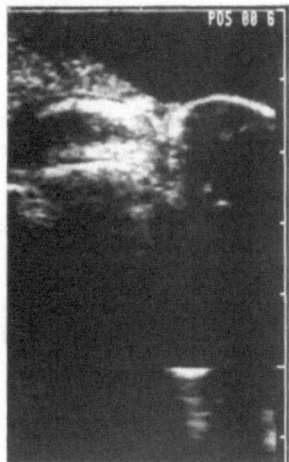

B

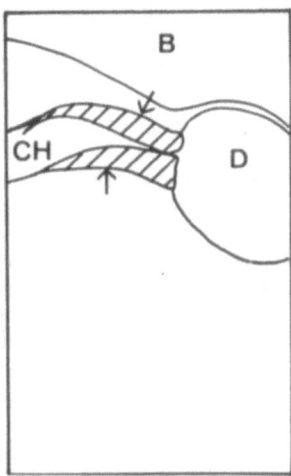

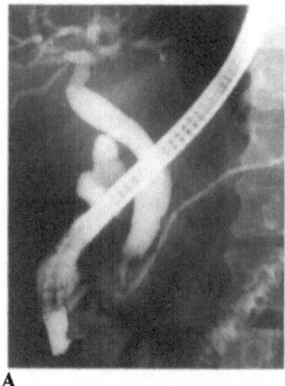

C

Figure 6.24.

A) ERCP in a patient with *obstructive jaundice:* presence of malignant stricture at the lower end of the common bile duct.

B) Intraoperative ultrasound in the same patient: oblique scan of the bilio-pancreatic ductal junction, with an interposed water-filled balloon (B) on the posterior surface of the pancreatic head: presence of a thickened wall of the lower part of the common bile duct (CH) at its entrance into the duodenum (D).

C) Surgical specimen of pancreato-duoden-ectomy in the same patient: excellent anatomical correlation between pathological findings and ultrasonographic image.

122

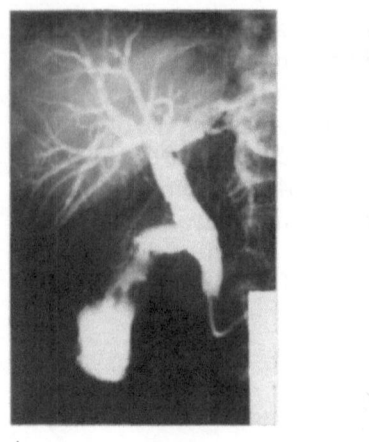 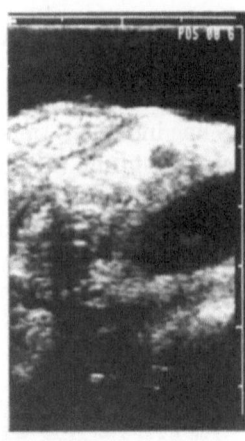 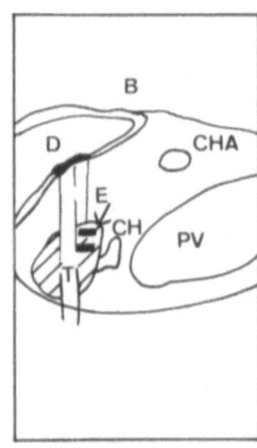

A   **B**

Figure 6.25. Patient operated for *obstructive jaundice* with dilatation of intra and extrahepatic bile ducts:
A) Obstruction of the distal part of the common bile duct on this preoperative ERCP, with a normal wirsungography: suspicion of primary cholangiocarcinoma.
B) Transverse scan of the head of the pancreas: in the distal part of the choledochus (CH), on the right side of the portal vein (PV), presence of a hypoechogenic tumor (T) with an excentric growth through the lumen of the choledochus occupied by an endoprosthesis (E).
The ultrasonic diagnosis of biliary obstruction is primary pancreatic adenocarcinoma, confirmed by surgical specimen of the pancreato-duodenectomy. Duodenum (D) with air bubbles giving artefacts. Common hepatic artery (CHA).

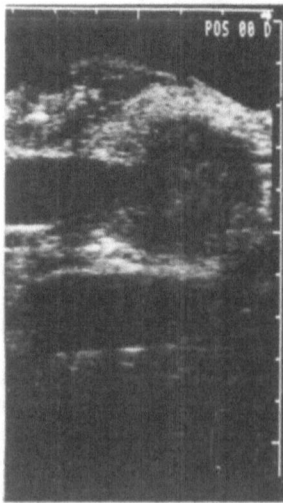 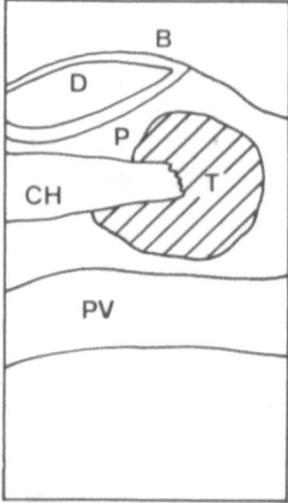

Fig. 6.26. Patient operated for obstructive jaundice.
Longitudinal scan showing an obliteration of the distal end of the common bile duct (CH) due to the presence of an hypoechoic mass (T) in the head of the pancreas. This picture is consistent with the diagnosis of cancer of the head of the pancreas.

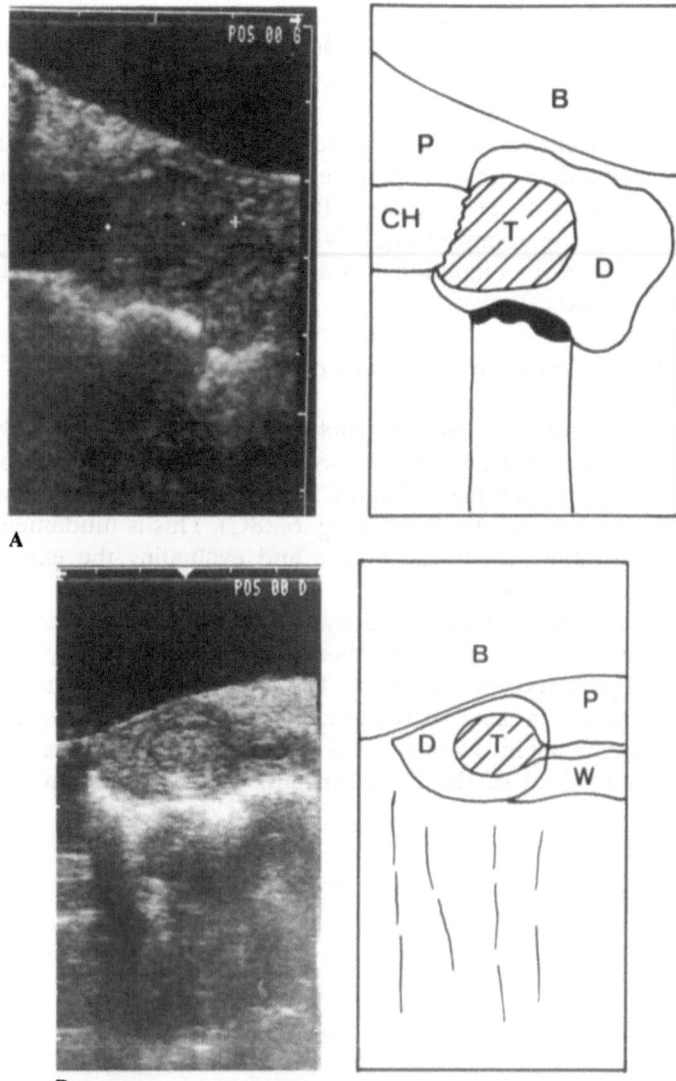

A

B

Figure 6.27. Patient operated for *obstructive jaundice* with dilatation of the intra and the extra-hepatic bile ducts and the Wirsung duct. No tumoral process detected on preoperative ultra-sound and CT-scanning. Normal preoperative gastroscopy.

A) Sagittal scan of the pancreatic head with an interposed water-filled balloon (B): obstruction of the distal part of the choledochus (CH), in the pancreatic head (P) by a tumoral process (T) protruding into the lumen of the duodenum (D). Ultrasonic diagnosis of tumor of the ampulla of Vater.

B) Transverse scan of the head of the pancreas (P), through a water-filled balloon (B). Obstruction of the dilated wirsung duct (W) by a small tumoral process (T), protruding into the lumen of the duodenum (D).

Confirmation of 15 mm malignant tumor of the ampulla of Vater on the surgical specimen of pancreato-duodenectomy.

Preoperative cholangiographic diagnostic methods (ERCP, PTC...) show indirect signs of a 'tumoral mass' which is ill defined on morphologic pre-operative examinations (US, CT-scan) because of its small size and infiltrative pattern. In our experience, the tumoral mass at the hilum is demonstrated 4 times out of 16 by ultrasound, and 8 times out of 16 by CT-scan examination. The common bile duct tumor is detected in 1 out of 4 US examinations as well as CT-scanning. In every case, IOUS detects the biliary tumor at the hilum or lower in the common duct. When there is a gallbladder tumor involving the main bile duct junction, it is detected in 4 out of 6 patients by both US examination and CT-scan.

2. Hepatic parenchymal invasion by bile duct tumors

The invasion of segment IV liver parenchymal tissue in gallbladder cancers is frequent, easily demonstrated by IOUS (Fig. 6.28B) and often previously demonstrated by preoperative US and CT-scan. Small size hepatic metastases can also be demonstrated by IOUS (Fig. 6.28C). This is fundamental in deciding the resectability of these tumors and evaluating the extent of liver resection to be performed.

In our experience, hepatic parenchymal invasion in gallbladder cancers involving the main bile duct junction is always demonstrated by IOUS but in only 4 out of 7 patients on preoperative US and CT-scan examination.

In the primary cholangiocarcinoma of the hilum (Klatskin tumors), posterior parenchymal invasion at the level of the caudate lobe is important in establishing the extent of the resection and can also be demonstrated by

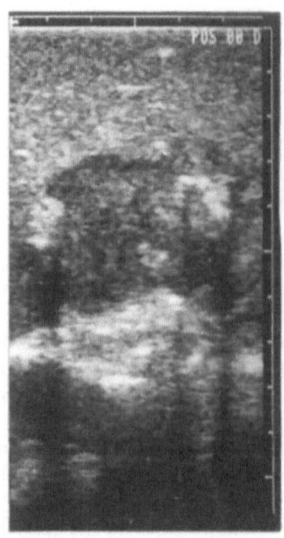
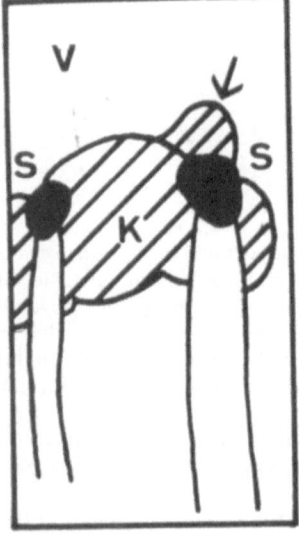

A

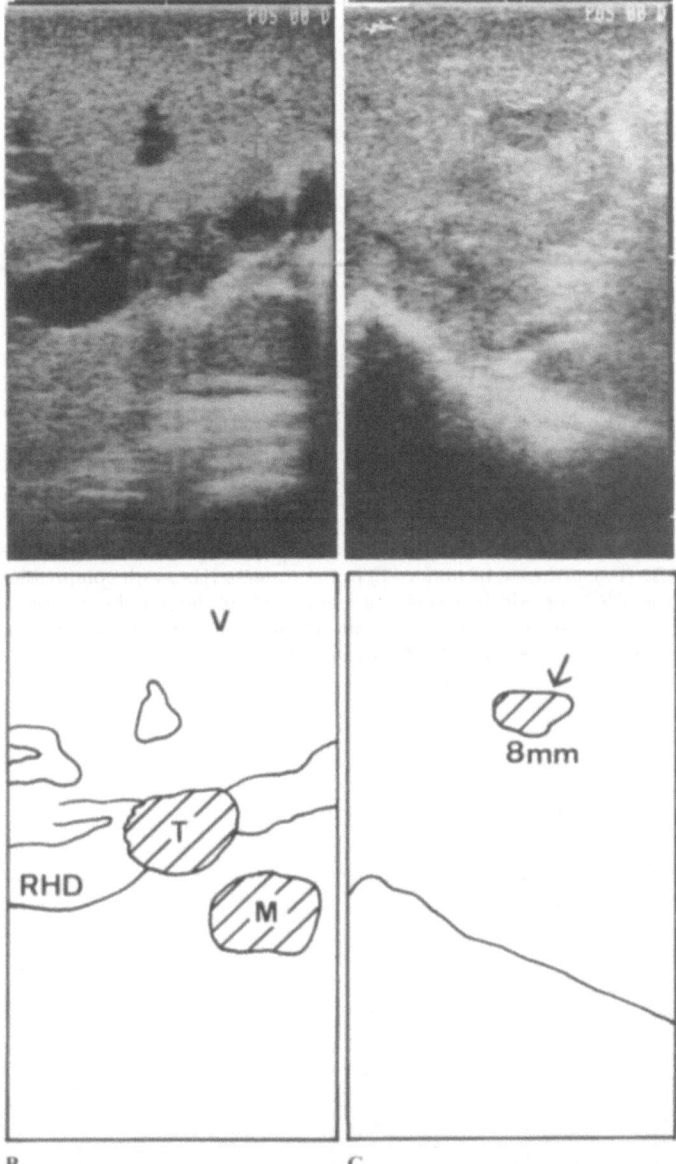

Figure 6.28. Patient operated for an *obstructive jaundice* with dilatation of the intra-hepatic bile ducts.

A) Transverse scan of the junction between segment IV and V on IOUS: the gallbladder is replaced by a diffuse tumoral process (K), associated with gallstones (S). Extension of the cancer (←) to the liver parenchyma of segment V.

B) Same patient: extension of the tumor into liver parenchyma (M) and invasion of the right biliary duct (T).

C) Presence of a small liver metastasis.

126

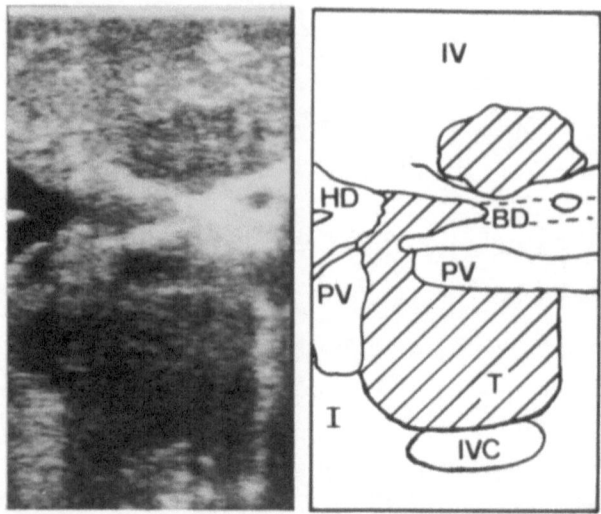

Figure 6.29. Sagittal scan of the biliary convergence, through the anterior surface of segment IV of COUINAUD (IV): presence of tumor (T) in the caudate lobe, with compression of the inferior vena cava (IVC) posteriorly and invasion anteriorly of the portal convergence (PV) and the biliary convergence, with dilatation of the intrahepatic bile duct (HD). Anteriorly, invasion of the liver parenchyma of segment IV of Couinaud (IV).

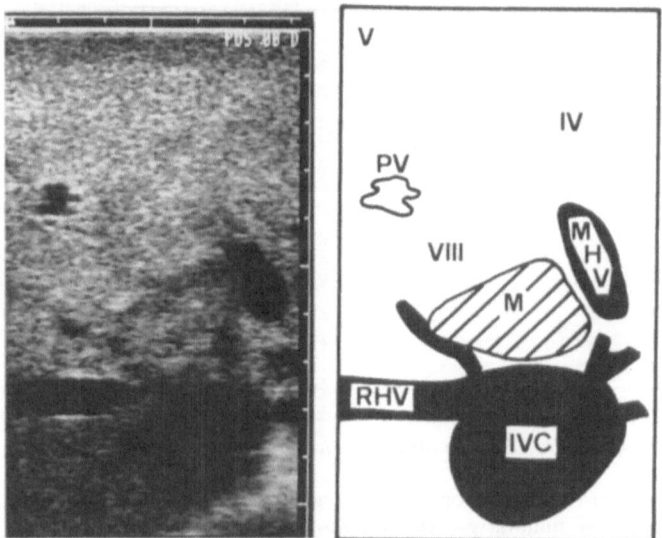

Figure 6.30. Intraoperative ultrasound: presence of an *occult liver metastasis* – confirm by echoguided biopsy – deeply sited in segment VIII of Couinaud (VIII) extending inferiorly into segment I, in correlation with the inferior vena cava (IVC), the middle hepatic vein (MHV) and the right hepatic vein (RHV). Histological diagnosis confirmed by an echoguided biopsy. Intraoperative palpation was normal.

IOUS (Fig. 6.29). Sagittal scanning of the hilum demonstrates the invasion of the caudate lobe on the posterior aspect of the tumor, which necessitates the resection of this part of the liver. Nevertheless, at the hilum, the infiltrative pattern of primary bile duct tumors and thus their ill defined contours, make it difficult to establish this diagnosis.

3. Liver and lymph node metastases

When there is substantial dilatation of the intrahepatic bile ducts, it is often difficult to detect the parenchymal metastases (Fig. 6.30). In one of our patients, these metastases were detected only after decompression of the bile ducts (Fig. 6.31). An echoguided biopsy is mandatory in assessing the pathology of these hypoechogenic tumoral masses.

In our experience, in 10 patients suffering from bile duct cancer with liver metastases, the sensitivity of preoperative ultrasound was 30%, while it was 40% for CT-Scan and 20% for arteriography. During surgery 70% of the metastases were partially palpable. IOUS always makes the diagnosis of these lesions possible, demonstrating the presence of occult hepatic metastases, half of which had not been detected on preoperative investigations.

Lymph node invasion, present in 14 of our patients, had never been correctly detected by preoperative US (1/14), CT-scan (1/14) or even by IOUS 85/14). In our experience, we found that no morphologic criteria are available to establish the difference between inflammatory and neoplastic lymph nodes. The diagnostic criteria based on echographic features or size are of no

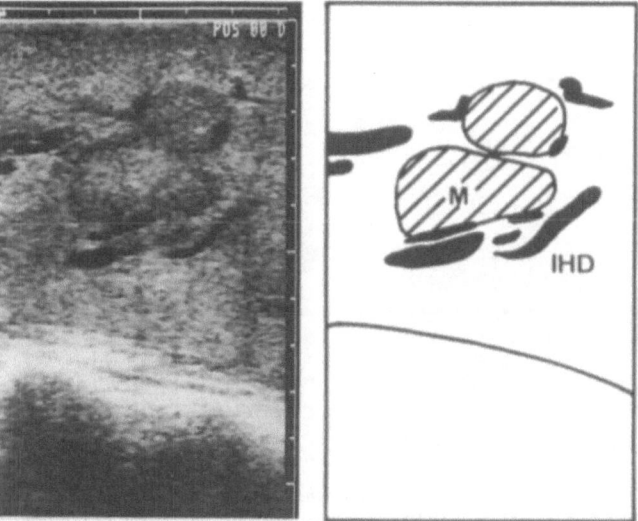

Figure 6.31. Patient operated for an *obstructive jaundice with hilar cancer.* Marked dilatation of the intrahepatic bile ducts leading to a difficult intra-operative ultrasonic examination of the liver parenchyma. After biliary decompression (IHD), detection of multiple liver metastases.

value. Accordingly, we do not routinely, during an exploratory laparotomy, look for lymph node invasion by IOUS but we start the operative procedure by removing them for immediate pathologic examination.

4. Vascular invasion

Vascular invasion, especially portal, is an important factor in determining the resectability of the tumor, the diagnosis of which necessitates an extensive dissection of the hilum: IOUS can detect this during an exploratory laparotomy without any dissection of the hilum or hepato-duodenal ligament structures.

On the contrary, such dissection is the cause of air artefacts which can prevent correct ultrasonic examination.

Nevertheless, before it is decided that resection is not possible on the basis of IOUS, one should apply strict criteria of vascular involvement: disappearance of the interface between the tumor and the external aspect of the venous wall (Figs. 6.32–6.33), intraluminal tumoral invasion of the vessel (Fig. 6.34) or presence of a portal thrombosis shown as a filling of the portal lumen by the tumor mass. In our experience, the pathologic correlation between surgical dissection of the hilum and IOUS in 14 patients with portal invasion demonstrates a sensitility of preoperative examination of 7% (1/14) for US, 29% (4/14) for CT-scan, 29% for arteriography and 21% (3/14) for Doppler-ultrasound. IOUS can detect vascular involvement in 93% (13/14) of cases, before surgical dissection which, of course, always detects this invasion.

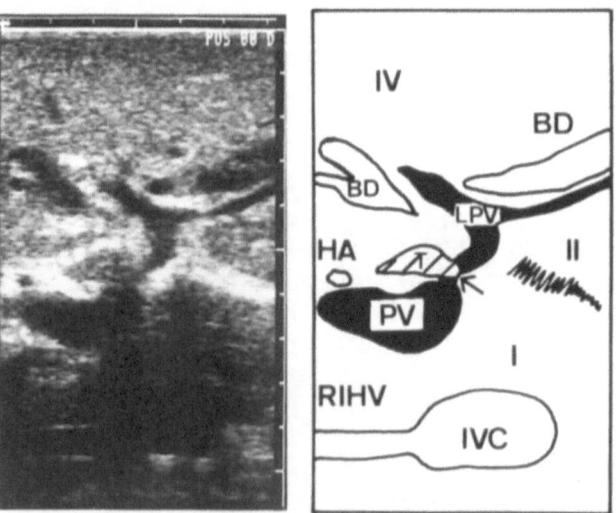

Figure 6.32. Transverse scan of the left side of the hepatic hilum in a patient with hilar cancer. The origin of the left portal vein (LPV) is narrowed by hilar tumor (T). Dilatation of the segmental biliary ducts (BD) of segment III and IV. Portal convergence (PV). Transverse scan of the hepatic artery (HA). Posteriorly, liver parenchyma of segment I and inferior vena cava (IVC), with a right inferior hepatic vein (RIHV).

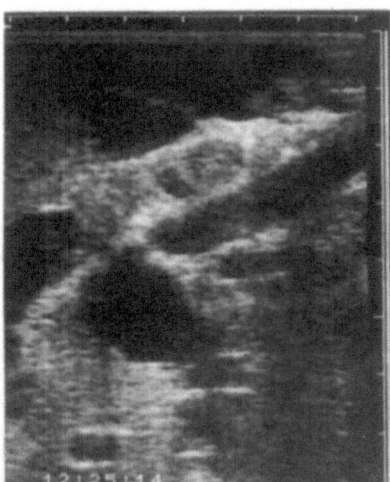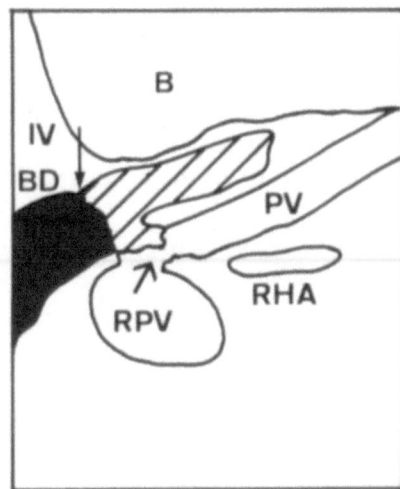

Figure 6.33. Sagittal scan of the hepatic duct at the level of biliary convergence, through an interposed water-filled balloon (B): obstruction (←) of the hepatic duct (BD) by a tumoral process invading (←) the junction between the portal vein (PV) and the right portal vein (RPV). Posteriorly, presence of a right hepatic artery (RHA).

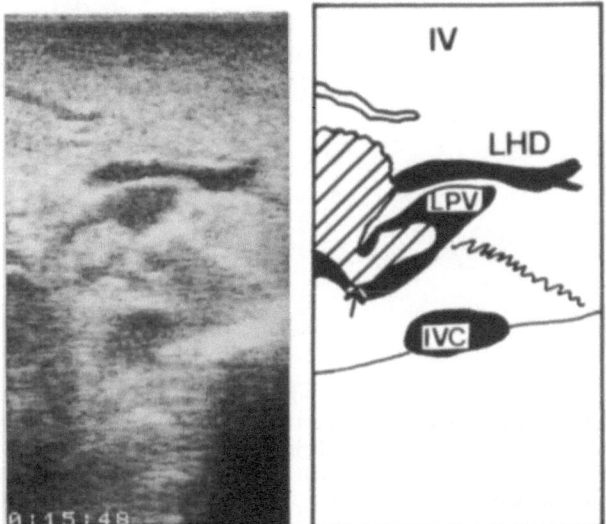

Figure 6.34. Transverse scan on the left side of the hepatic hilum: the left hepatic duct (LHD) is interrupted by an ill-defined isoechogenic tumor (T) with posterior invasion of the left portal vein by a neoplastic thrombus (←). Posteriorly, inferior vena cava (IVC). Liver parenchyma of segment I, II and IV.
With permission of Acta Gastro-Enterologica Belgica (18).

Two different features have to be distinguished:
1. Complete portal thrombosis (7 patients) (Fig. 6.35) is often diagnosed before the operation by Doppler-ultrasound (3/4), arteriography (4/6), and CT-scanning (4/7). IOUS always detects the thrombosis 7/7) prior to any surgical dissection (7/7).
2. Partial invasion of the venous wall (7 patients) without thrombosis is never

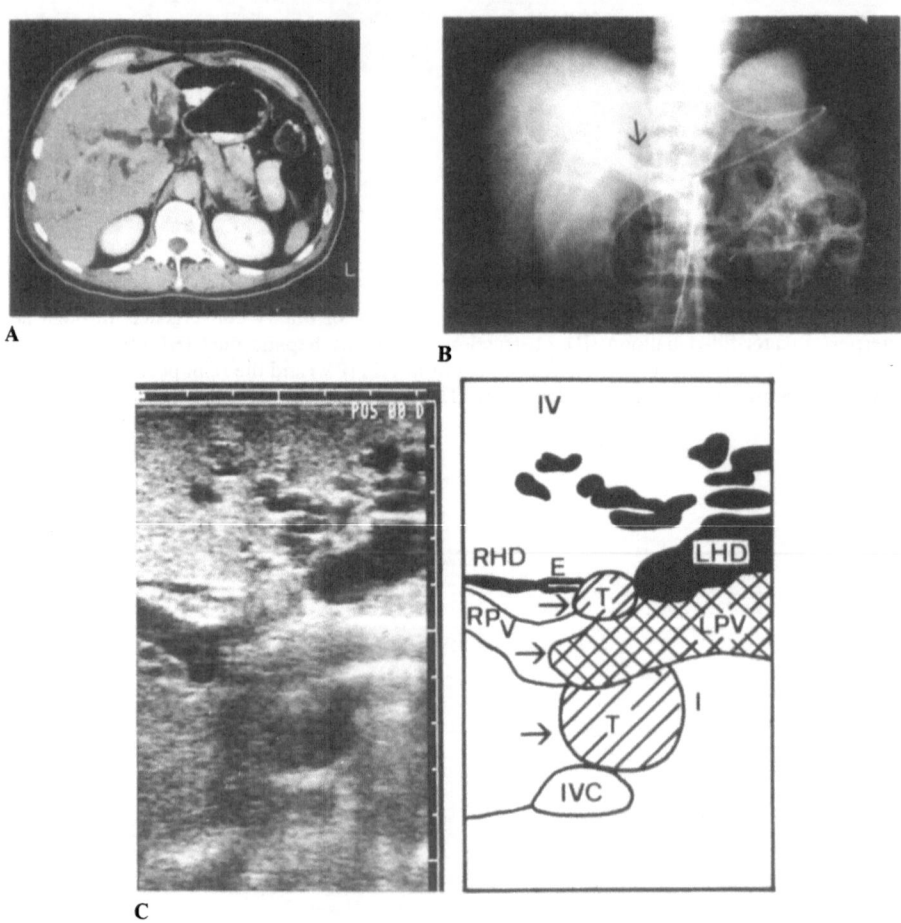

Figure 6.35. Patient with obstructive jaundice and dilatation of the intra and extrahepatic bile ducts: complete obstruction of the hepatic duct at the biliary convergence on preoperative ERCP. Insertion of an endoprosthesis in the right intrahepatic bile duct.

A) CT-scan of the hepatic hilum: dilatation of left and right intrahepatic ducts. Patent right portal vein. No visualization of the left portal vein.

B) Preoperative arteriogram: obstruction of the left portal vein (→).

C) Intraoperative ultrasound: transverse scan of the hepatic hilum. Dilated left intra-hepatic duct (LHD) and presence of the prosthesis (E) in a non dilated right hepatic duct (RHD). Posteriorly, portal convergence with a normal right portal vein (RPV) and presence of a thrombus (→) in the left portal vein (LPV). Tumoral process (T) sited in segment I of Couinaud (I) invading cranially the portal and the biliary convergence (→). Inferior vena cava (IVC).

diagnosed by preoperative examination: Doppler-ultrasond (0/6), arteriography (0/4), CT-scan (0/7), while IOUS will show this mural invasion on 6 out of 7 patients (86%); the last patient, who had an extended right hepatectomy performed for a tumor of the hilum already treated by an endoprosthesis for 6 months, had a microscopic invasion of the wall of the right portal branch which appeared macroscopically normal.

It should be noted that, during the operation, partial vascular invasion is always detected at the endstage of the dissection of the hilum and therefore IOUS is most useful in supplying additional information to preoperative investigations: this was the case in our prospective series of 27 patients (14 of them (52%) demonstrating local spread: invasion of the parenchyma, liver metastasis, portal invasion). This information proved decisive for resectability in patients (40%) and in evaluating resectability in 11 patients (40%).

During the operation for tumor of the bile ducts, IOUS can be helpful for palliative procedures: when there is an invasion of the intrahepatic bile ducts at the level of their secondary convergence, IOUS permits intraoperative echoguided cholangiography via puncture of the anatomically excluded segments of the liver. After decompression of the bile ducts by bilio-digestive anastomosis or trans-tumoral intubation, IOUS can eventually demonstrate the lack of drainage of these same excluded segments and indicate when complementary drainage must be performed. For three patients with a non-resectable hilar tumor, bilateral drainage was performed during exploratory laparotomy by implanting an echoguided trans-tumoral prosthesis (Fig. 6.36).

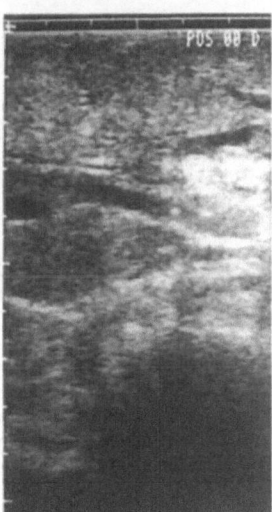 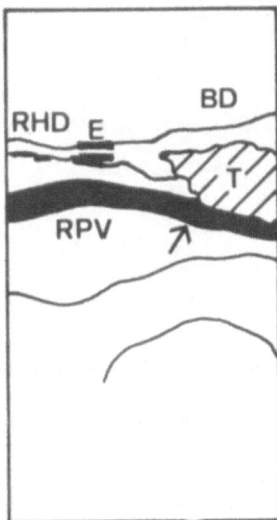

Figure 6.36. Transverse scan at the right side of the hepatic hilum: hyperechogenic hilar tumor (T) obstructing the biliary convergence (BD) and the anterior wall (←) of the right portal vein (RPV).
Intraoperatively, we performed under ultrasound – guidance, a transtumoral intubation (E) of the tumoral obstruction (T) through the right hepatic duct (RHD).

132

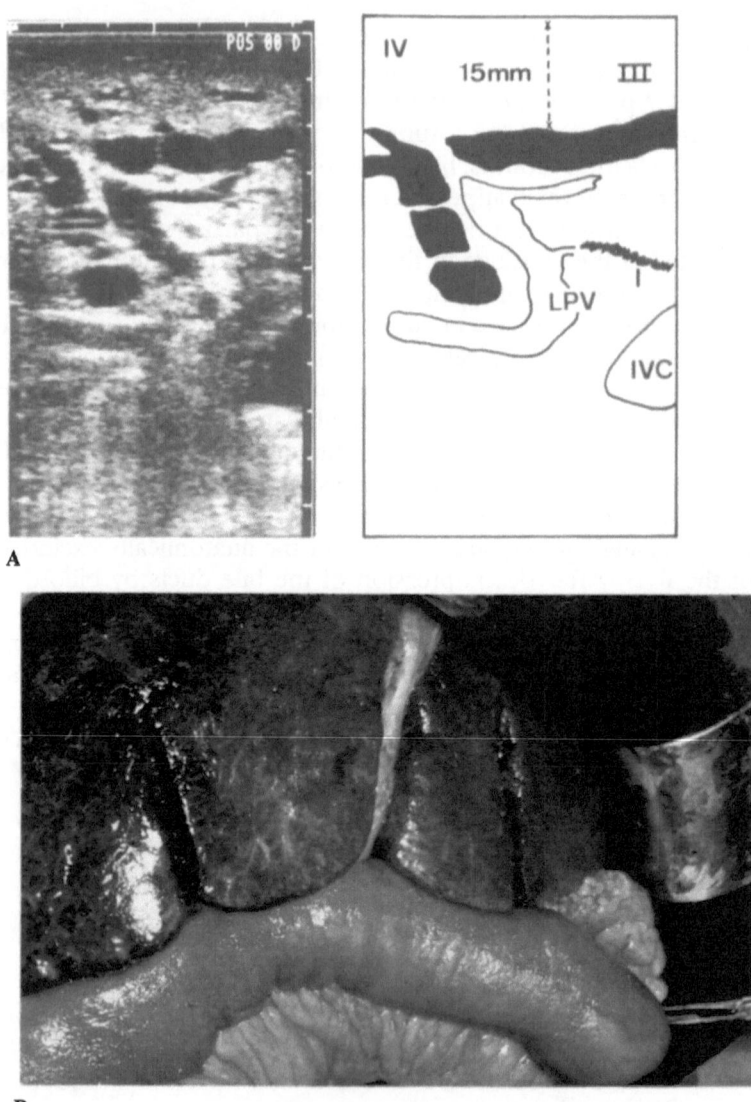

A

B

Figure 6.37. Patient operated for *cancer of the hepatic hilum invading the secondary biliary convergences:*
A) Transverse scan at the left side of the hepatic hilum: dilatation of the left hepatic duct and the segmental bile ducts of segment III of Couinaud, above the left portal vein (LPV) and the segmental portal vein of segment III. Distance of 15 mm between the liver surface and the segmental bile duct of segment III.
B) Bilateral peripheric intrahepatic cholangio-anastomoses on the segmental bile duct of segment III and segmental bile duct of segment V.

Palliative bilio-digestive anastomosis employing segment III bile duct is well known [6, 12]. However, IOUS can be helpful in finding the segmental bile duct and measuring its distance from the liver capsule (Fig. 6.37A). Moreover, IOUS can detect segment V bile duct, the location of which is more variable and can thus be used for a right intrahepatic bilio-digestive anastomosis. For two patients with a non resectable hilar tumor, invading the secondary biliary convergence, right and left peripheral intrahepatic bilio-digestive anastómoses have been possible by the use of IOUS (Fig. 6.37B). Echoguided puncture of the bile ducts can be performed for intraoperative cholangiography with a reduced risk of hemobilia, even in poorly dilated intra-hepatic segmental ducts. Echoguided biopsies of bile duct tumors or suspect hepatic nodules can also be performed, permitting an accurate histological diagnosis.

IOUS is a fundamental investigation during exploratory laparotomy for bile duct cancer. It can evidence local spread of cancer of the hilum giving decisive information on resectability prior to any surgical dissection.

Conclusions

For biliary stones, IOUS is of interest in diagnosing gallbladder microlithiasis or when a preoperative work-up has not be done (emergency operations, non biliary operations such as colon surgery or cirrhosis) or has not been satisfactory (morbid obesity). In common duct lithiasis, the detection power of IOUS is on the whole comparable to intraoperative cholangiography: combined use of both techniques reduces to a great extent negative choledocotomies and residual stones and this constitute progress in this kind of surgery necessitating complete removal of the stones. Each technique has its specific advantages and drawbacks. For intrahepatic lithiasis, IOUS is useful in the detection and precise anatomical localization of the stones. It can also improve treatment modalities: echoguided removal of the stones, intubation, bile duct dilatation by tubes or balloons and hepatotomies. If hepatectomy is needed, it can indicate the exact limits of the resection according to the extent of the lithiasis.

For tumor of the bile ducts, IOUS can be helpful in diagnosis by precisely localizing the tumor and its spread within the ducts. Regional invasion (liver metastases, parenchymal and vascular involvement) is detected by IOUS before any extensive surgical dissection, particularly in cases of cancer of the hilum. IOUS can also be of value in its treatment since knowledge of the local extension of this cancer is fundamental in assessing its resectability. Liver metastases can be confirmed by echoguided biopsies, an echoguided puncture of the bile ducts is useful in performing selective cholangiography, transtumoral intubation or bile duct drainage. Intrahepatic peripheral cholangio-anastomoses can be performed thanks to ultrasound localization of the dilated duct beneath the surface of the liver parenchyma.

134

Acknowledgement

We wish to thank Miss Michele Lemaire, Mr. Luc Iweins, Dr. Benoit Lengelé for the illustrations, Mrs. Nadine Thiebaut for typing the manuscript and Miss Therese O'Connor for the English translation.

References

1. Adson M., Nagorney D.: *Hepatic resection for intrahepatic ductal stones.* Arch. Surg. 117: 611–616, 1982.
2. Belghiti J., Menu Y.: *Echographie peropératoire dans le traitement de la lithiase intrahépatique.* J.E.M.U. 8: 2–3, 97–98, 1987.
3. Bismuth H., Castaing D.: *Le traitement chirurgical de la lithiase de la voie biliaire principale.* Chirurgie 109: 353–356, 1983.
4. Bismuth H., Castaing D.: *Echographie peropératoire du foie et des voies biliaires.* Flammarion, Médecine-Sciences, Paris, 1985.
5. Bismuth H., Castaing D., Traynor O.: *Resection or palliation: priority of surgery in the treatment of hilar cancer.* World J. Surg. 12: 39–47, 1988.
6. Bismuth H., Corlette M. B.: *Intrahepatic cholangioenteric anastomosis in carcinoma of the hilus of the liver.* Surg. Gyn. & Obst. 140: 170–178, 1975.
7. Blumgart L. J., Benjamin I. S., Hadjis N. S., Beazley R.: *Surgical approaches to cholangiocarcinoma at confluence of hepatic ducts.* Lancet, 66–69, 1984.
8. Chardavoyne R., Kumari-Subhaya S., Auguste L. J., Phillips G., Stein T. A., Wise L.: *Comparison of intra-operative ultrasonography and cholangiography in detection of small common bile duct stones.* Ann. Surg. 206: 1, 53–55, 1987.
9. Choi T., Wong J., Ong G. B.: *The surgical management of primary intrahepatic stones.* Br. J. Surg. 69: 86–90, 1982.
10. Choi T., Wong J.: *Partial hepatectomy for intrahepatic stones.* World J. Surg. 10: 281–286, 1986.
11. Collier N. A., Carr D., Hemingway A., Blumgart L. H.: *Preoperative diagnosis and its effect on the treatment of carcinoma of the gallbladder.* Surg. Gyn. Obst. 159: 465–470, 1984.
12. Couinaud M. C.: *Cholangio-jéjunostomies intrahépatiques gauches. A propos de 18 observations personnelles.* Archives Françaises des Maladies de l'Appareil Digestif 56: 4, 295–310, 1967.
13. Denbensten L., Doty J. E.: *Pathogenesis and management of choledecolithiasis.* Surg. Clin. North. Am. 61: 893–907, 1981.
14. Denbenstein L., Berci G.: *The current status of biliary tract surgery: an international study of 1072 consecutive patients.* World J. Surg. 10: 116–122, 1986.
15. Eiseman B., Greenlaw R. H., Gallagher J. Q.: *Localisation of common duct stones by ultrasound.* Arch. Surg. 91: 195–199, 1965.
16. Escat J., Fourtanier G., Maigne C., Fournier D.: *Notre expérience de la cholédocotomie pour lithiase.* Chirurgie 109: 471–473, 1983.
17. Espinoza P., Kunstlinger F., Liguory C., Meduri B., Pelleltier G., Etienne J. P.: *Valeur de l'échotomographie pour le diagnostic de lithiase de la voie biliaire principale.* Gastroenterol. Clin. Biol. 8: 42–46, 1984.
18. Evander A., Fredlund P., Hoevels J., Ihse I., Bengmark S.: *Evaluation of aggressive surgery for carcinoma of the extrahepatic bile ducts.* Ann. Surg. 191: 1, 23–29, 1980.
19. Gibson R. N., Yeung E., Thompson J. N., Carr D. H., Hemingway A. P., Bradpiece H. A., Benjamin I. S., Blumgart L. H., Allison D. J.: *Bile duct obstruction: radiologic evaluation of level, cause, and tumor resectability.* Radiology 160: 43–47, 1986.

135

20. Gigot J. F., Lambert F., Warzee P., Pringot J., Mathurin P., Otte J. B. and Kestens P. J.: *Démarches diagnostiques et thérapeutiques dans les cancers du hile: expérience U.C.L.* M.C.D. 16: 10–11, 1987.
21. Gigot J. F., Puttemans T., Gianello P., Dardenne A. N., Detry R., Otte J. B. et Kestens P. J.: *L'échographie peropératoire en chirurgie hépato-biliaire: résultats préliminaires.* Acta Gastro-Enterologica Belgica 4: 434–446, 1985.
22. Gigot J. F., Detry R., Dardenne A. N., Pringot J., Otte J. B. et Kestens P. J.: *Apport de l'échographie peropératoire en chirurgie pancréatique: à propos de 63 patients.* J.E.M.U. 8: 2–3, 123–129, 1987.
23. Gigot J. F., Geubel A., Dardenne A. N., Goncette L. and Kestens P. J.: *Le rôle de l'échographie peropératoire dans la chirurgie biliaire lithiasique: résultats préliminaires.* Acta Gastro-Enterologica Belgica (in press).
24. Glenn F.: *Trends in surgical treatment of calculus disease of the biliary tract.* Surg. Gyn. Obstr. 140: 877–884, 1975.
25. Gozzetti G., Mazziotti A., Bolondi L.: *Echografia intraoperatoria in chirurgia epato-biliare e pancreatica.* Masson Italia Editori – Milano – 1986.
26. Hall R. C., Sakaiyazak P., Kim S. K. and all: *Failure of operative cholangiography to prevent retained common duct stones.* Am. J. Surg. 125: 51–57, 1973.
27. Hayashi S., Wagai T., Miyazawa R., Ito K., Ischikawa S., Uematsu K., Kikuchi Y., Uchida R.: *Ultrasonic diagnosis of breast tumor and cholelithiasis.* West. J. Surg., Obst. Gynec. 70: 34–40, 1962.
28. Herbst C. A., Mittelstaedt C. A., Staab, E. V., Buckwalter J. A.: *Intraoperative ultrasonography evaluation of the gall bladder in morbidly obese patients.* Ann. Surg. 200: 6, 691–692, 1984.
29. Iwasaki Y., Okamura T., Ozaki A., Todoroki T., Takase Y., Ohara K., Nishimura A., Otsu H.: *Surgical treatment for carcinoma at the confluence of the major hepatic ducts.* Surg. Gyn. Obst. 162: 457–464, 1986.
30. Jakimowicz J. J., Carol E. J., Jurgens P. T. H. J.: *The peroperative use of real-time B-mode ultrasound imaging in biliary and pancreatic surgery.* Dig. Surg. 1: 55–60, 1984.
31. Jakimovicz J. J., Rutten H., Jurgens P. J., Carol E. J.: *Comparison of operative ultrasonography and radiography in screening of the common bile duct for calculi.* World J. Surg. 11: 628–634, 1987.
32. Kakos G. S., Tompkins R. K., Turnipseed W., Zollinger R. M.: *Operative cholangiography during routine cholecystectomy: review of 3012 cases.* Arch. Surg. 104: 484–488, 1972.
33. Knight P. R., Newell J. A.: *Operative use of ultrasonics in cholelithiasis.* Lancet, 1023–1025, 1963.
34. Kunstlinger F., Castaing D., Houssin D. et Bismuth H.: *Diagnostic échographique des lithiases intrahépatiques.* Gastro-Enterol. Clin. Biol. 8: 122–125, 1984.
35. Lane R. J., Crocker E. F.: *Operative ultrasonic bile duct scanning.* Aust. N. Z. Surg. 49: 4, 454–458, 1979.
36. Lane R. J., Glazer G.: *Intraoperative B-mode ultrasound scanning of the extra-hepatic biliary system and pancreas.* Lancet, 334–337, 1980.
37. Lane R. J., Coupland G. A. E.: *Ultrasonic indications to explore the common bile duct.* Surgery 91: 3, 268–274, 1982.
38. Langer J. C., Langer B., Taylor B. R., Zeldin R., Cummings B.: *Carcinoma of the extrahepatic bile ducts: results of an aggressive surgical approach.* Surgery 98: 4, 752–759, 1985.
39. Launois B., Campion J. P., Brissot P., Gosselin M.: *Carcinoma of the hepatic hilus: surgical management and the case for resection.* Ann. Surg. 190: 2, 151–157, 1979.
40. Machi J., Sigel B., Spigos D. G., Beitler J. C., Justine J. R.: *Experimental assessment of imaging variables associated with operative ultrasonic and radiographic cholangiography.* J. Ultrasound Med. 2: 535–538, 1983.
41. Machi J., Sigel B., Mc Grath E. C., Beitler J. C., Ramos J. R., Work B. A.: *Operative ultrasonography in the biliary tract during pregnancy.* Surg. Gyn. Obst. 160: 119–123, 1985.

136

42. Mizumoto R., Kawarada Y., Suzuki H.: *Surgical treatment of hilar carcinoma of the bile duct.* Surg. Gyn. Obst. 162: 153–158, 1986.
43. Mouiel J., Bus J. J., Bertrand J. C., Chabannes B., Ceccanti J. P., Giaume F.: *Le traitement chirurgical de la lithiase biliaire intrahépatique diffuse. Apport de la résection du segment IV et des hépatotomies guidées.* Ann. Chir. 32 (10): 739–744, 1978.
44. Nakayama F., Furusawa T., Nakama T.: *Hepatolithiasis in Japan: present status.* Am. J. Surg. 139: 216–220, 1980.
45. Okuda K., Ohto M., Tsuchiya Y.: *The role of ultrasound, percutaneous transhepatic cholangiography, computed tomographic scanning and magnetic resonance imaging in the preoperative assessment of bile duct cancer.* World J. Surg. 12: 18–26, 1988.
46. Pelissier E., Meyer J. M.: *Etude critique d'un milier d'interventions pour lithiase biliaire.* Chirurgie 108: 222–227, 1982.
47. Pichlmayr R., Ringe B., Lauchart W., Bechstein W., Gubernatis G., Wagner E.: *Radical resection and liver grafting as the two main components of surgical strategy in the treatment of proximal bile duct cancer.* World J. Surug. 12: 68–77, 1988.
48. Sakaguchi S., Nakamura S.: *Surgery of the portal vein in resection of cancer of the hepatic hilus.* Surgery 90: 3, 344–349, 1986.
49. Sato T., Suzuki N., Takahashi W., Unematsu I.: *Surgical management of intrahepatic gallstones.* Ann. Surg. 192: 1, 28–32, 1980.
50. Sigel B., Spigos D. G., Donahue P. E., Pearl R., Popky G. L., Nyhus L. M.: *Intraoperative ultrasonic visualisation of biliary calculi.* Current Surgery 36: 158–159, 1979.
51. Sigel B., Coelho J. C. U., Spigos D. G., Donahue P. E., Renigers S. A., Capek V., Nyhus L. M., Popky G. L.: *Real-time ultrasonography during biliary surgery.* Radiology 137: 531–533, 1980.
52. Sigel B., Coelho J. C. U., Spigos D. G., Donahue P. E., Wood D. K., Nyhus L. M.: *Ultrasonic imaging during biliary and pancreatic surgery.* Am. J. Surg. 141: 84–89, 1981.
53. Sigel B.: *Operative ultrasonography.* Lea and Fabinger, Philadelphia, 1982.
54. Sigel B., Coelho J. C. U., Nyhus L. M., Donahue P. E., Velasco J. M., Spigos D. G.: *Comparison of cholangiography and ultrasonography in the operative screening of the common bile duct.* World J. Surg. 6: 440–444, 1982.
55. Sigel B., Machi J., Beitler J. C., Donahue P. E., Bombeck C. T., Baker R. J., Duarte B.: *Comparative accuracy of operative ultrasonography and cholangiography in detecting common duct calculi.* Surgery 94: 4, 715–720, 1983.
56. Sigel B., Machi J., Kikushi T., Anderson K. W., Zaren H. A.: *Role of intraoperative ultrasound in biliary surgery.* J.E.M.U. 8: 2–3, 93–96, 1987.
57. Voyles C. R., Bowley N. J., Allison D. J., Benjamin I. S., Blumgart L. H.: *Carcinoma of the proximal extrahepatic biliary tree: radiologic assessment and therapeutic alternatives.* Ann. Surg. 197: 2, 188–194, 1983.
58. Way L. W., Admirand W. H., Dunphy J. E.: *Management of choledoco lithiasis.* Ann. Surg. 76: 347–359, 1972.
59. Williamson B. W. A., Blumgart L. H., McKellar N. J.: *Management of tumors of the liver: combined use of arteriography and venography in the assessment of resectability, especially in hilar tumors.* Am. J. Surg. 139: 210–215, 1980.

Chapter 7: Intraoperative ultrasound during pancreatic surgery

In surgery of the pancreas intraoperative ultrasound has three fields of application: cancer, chronic pancreatitis or pseudocysts and endocrine tumors. Intraoperative ultrasound not only establishes diagnosis in doubtful cases but also provides a clear idea of the location of lesions vis-à-vis the vascular structures – superior mesenteric vein and artery and portal vein – as well as evidencing any alterations to the pancreatic duct. Endocrine tumors, whose primary site is often difficult to identify despite the recent advances in diagnostics, can more often than not be readily visualized at intraoperative scan.

Exploration technique

The pancreas can be explored through the adjacent structures of the stomach, duodenum, and gastro-cholic ligament (Fig. 7.1), or by placing the probe directly on the surface of the gland after incision of the gastro-cholic ligament. In this case, a gel pad should be used as an interface between probe and organ so as to allow visualization of the superficial structures and avoid compression of the veins or pancreatic duct by the probe.

A linear array probe should be used. Both longitudinal and transverse scans must be taken for a complete picture of the gland and its vascular-

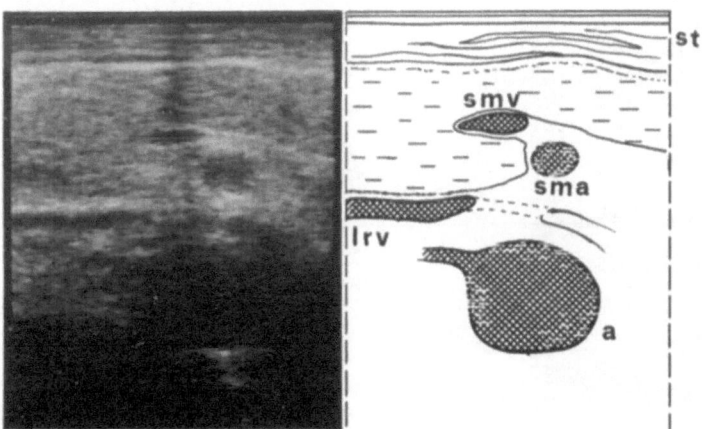

Figure 7.1. Normal pancreas. Transverse scan through the gastric wall clearly shows the uncinate process posterior to the superior mesenteric vein.

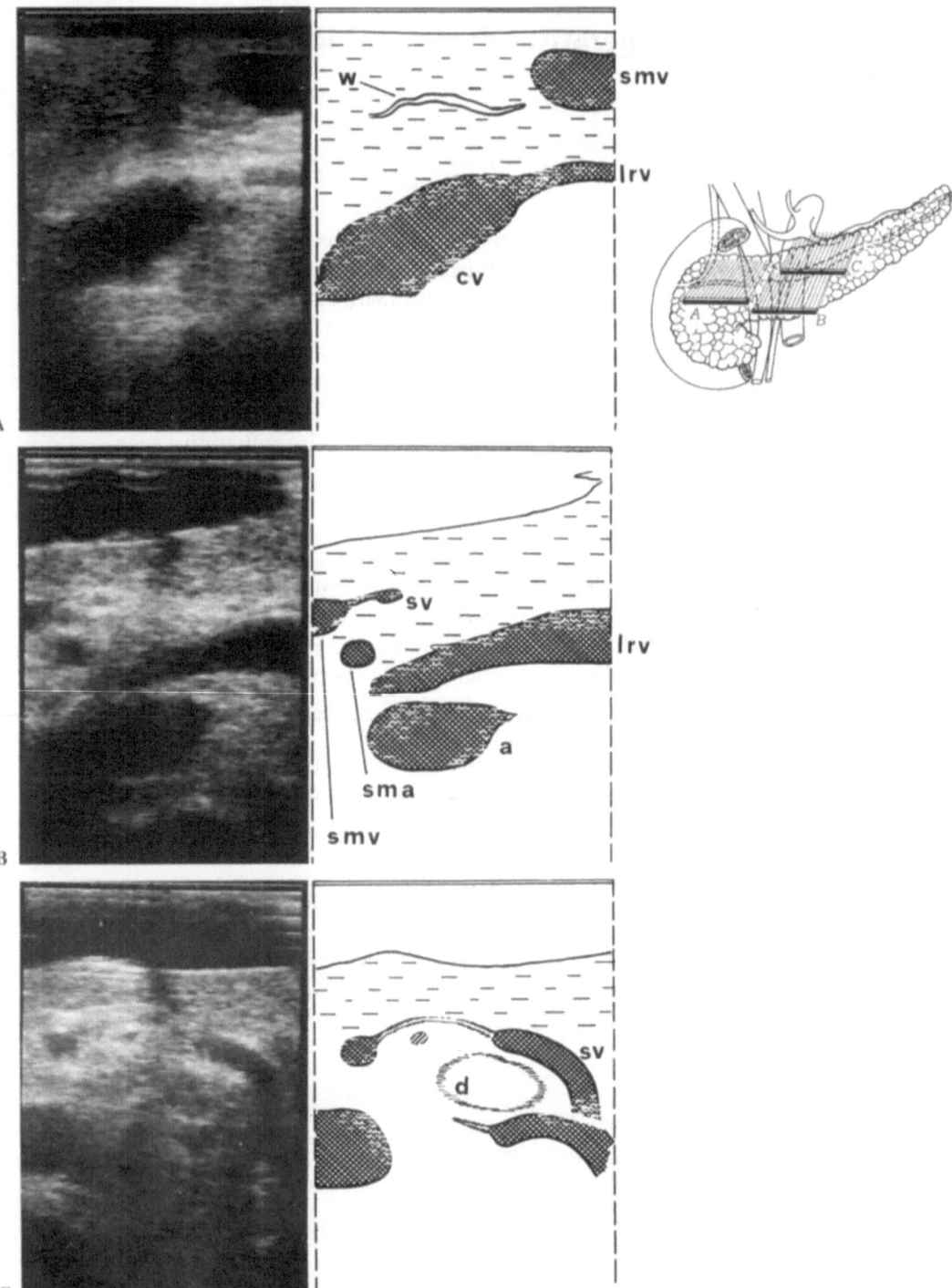

Figure 7.2. Normal pancreas.
A) Scan on a level with the head. Note the close proximity of both the vena cava and the superior mesenteric vein. A small segment of the Wirsung duct (w) is also visible.
B, C) Scan on a level with the body of the pancreas, using a gel cushion.

ductal apparatus. Longitudinal scans will show the superior mesenteric vein, the portal vein and the common bile duct, while transverse scans give good visualization of the Wirsung duct and the splenic vein. Both types of scan should be carried out for a true appreciation of the lesion and the extent to which it impinges upon adjacent tissue. This is especially true in the case of tumors of the head of the pancreas near the superior mesenteric vein.

The parenchyma of the head of the pancreas presents a regular, moderately echogenic appearance made up of fine, evenly distributed echoes of similar amplitude. This echo-pattern reflects the web of connective tissue and small pancreatic ducts in this area. Echogenicity is largely determined by the amount of lipid infiltration in the parenchyma, which varies with age and individual metabolism [8]. The pancreatic duct appears as a linear canal with sharply echogenic walls; diameter in this area is approximately 2 mm. Also clearly visible is the common bile duct and on occasion, the papilla of Vater can be detected among the duodenal villi. Shifting the probe medially to the junction between the head and body of the pancreas, the superior mesenteric vein appears surrounded by the caudate process. 3–5 mm lateral to this and below the vein, runs the superior mesenteric artery (between vein and aorta) and which is about one third the size of the vein. In this area the pancreas is less thick, being about 1.2–1.7 cm. On transverse scan the splenic vein appears very clearly as it courses the length of the body to the tail of the pancreas. This caudate area may be less readily visualized since it extends posteriorly up to the hilum of the spleen (Fig. 7.2).

Pancreatic carcinomas

Once again intraoperative ultrasound during surgery for tumors of the exocrine pancreas is not only able to clinch diagnosis but allows the surgeon to visualize tumor extension and possible involvement of contiguous vessels – an all important fact that will weigh heavily in decision making.

Pancreatic carcinoma presents as a heterogeneous, poorly echoic mass with irregular contours on account of peripheral tumor digitation as well as the effect of beam attenuation [2, 8, 27, 32, 36] (Figs. 7.3, 7.4, 7.5). Cystic tumors – an infrequent finding – show up as irregularly echogenic with scattered hypoechoic or indeed anechoic lacunae (Fig. 7.6).

Although carcinomas and chronic pancreatitis do not present any specific differences at ultrasound, tumors tend to be less echoic than the nodules formed in pancreatitis, which tend to have heightened echogenicity. However, other conditions visible at ultrasound help to suggest cancer, namely bile duct obstruction [40], the extension of the pancreatic swelling (Fig. 7.7) and the appearance of a dilated Wirsung duct (Fig. 7.8) as well as stones in this duct. Echo-guided biopsy will dispel any remaining doubts. A typical appearance, present in 13 of our 19 patients with carcinoma of the head of the pancreas, is an irregular choledocal lumen caused by neoplastic infiltration or seeding

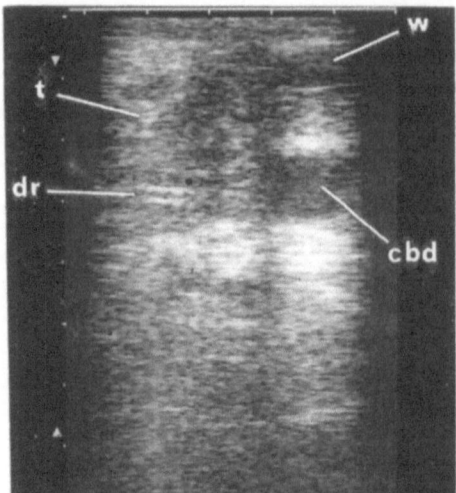

Figure 7.3. Pancreatic cancer. Inhomogeneous hypoechoic 3 cm lesion (t) in the head of the pancreas. Note its proximity to the Wirsung duct (w) (which appears dilated) and the common bile duct (cbd). Inside the tumor a 'railway track' appearance denotes transtumoral transhepatic drainage (dr).

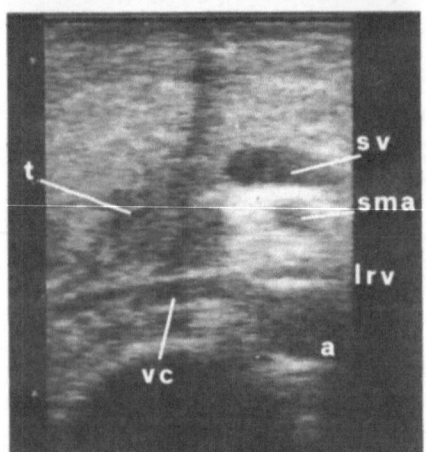

Figure 7.4. Neoplasm in the uncinate process shows as a mass of low-level echoes with irregular margins (A).
B) Operative specimen: cephaloduodenopancreatectomy.

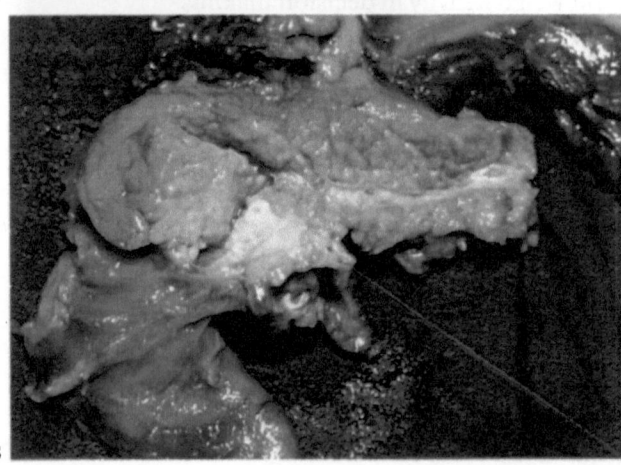

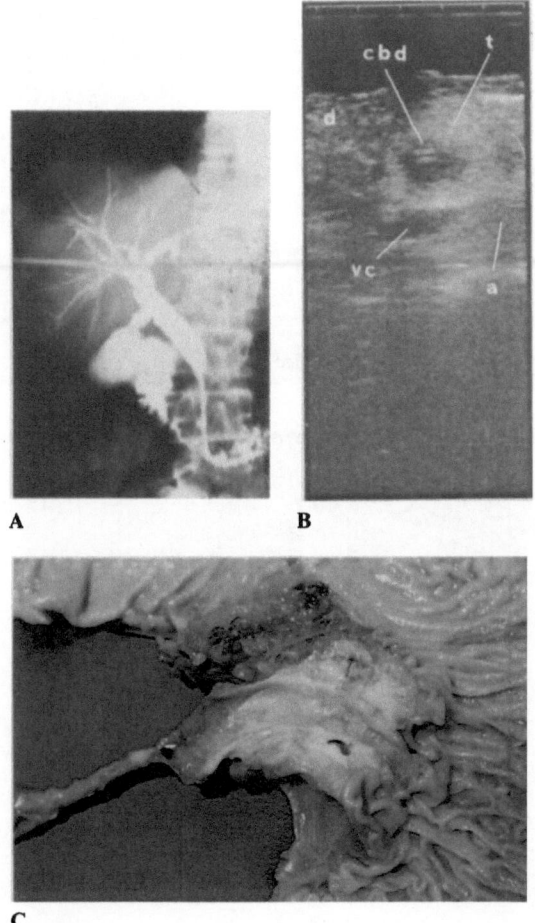

A   B

C

Figure 7.5. Neoplasmm of the head of the pancreas. A transhepatic, transtumoral catheter had been placed prior to surgery (A).

B) Tumor presents as a hyperechoic mass through which runs a dilated bile duct and the 'railway track' image of the catheter.

C) Operative piece: cephalduodenopancreatectomy.

142

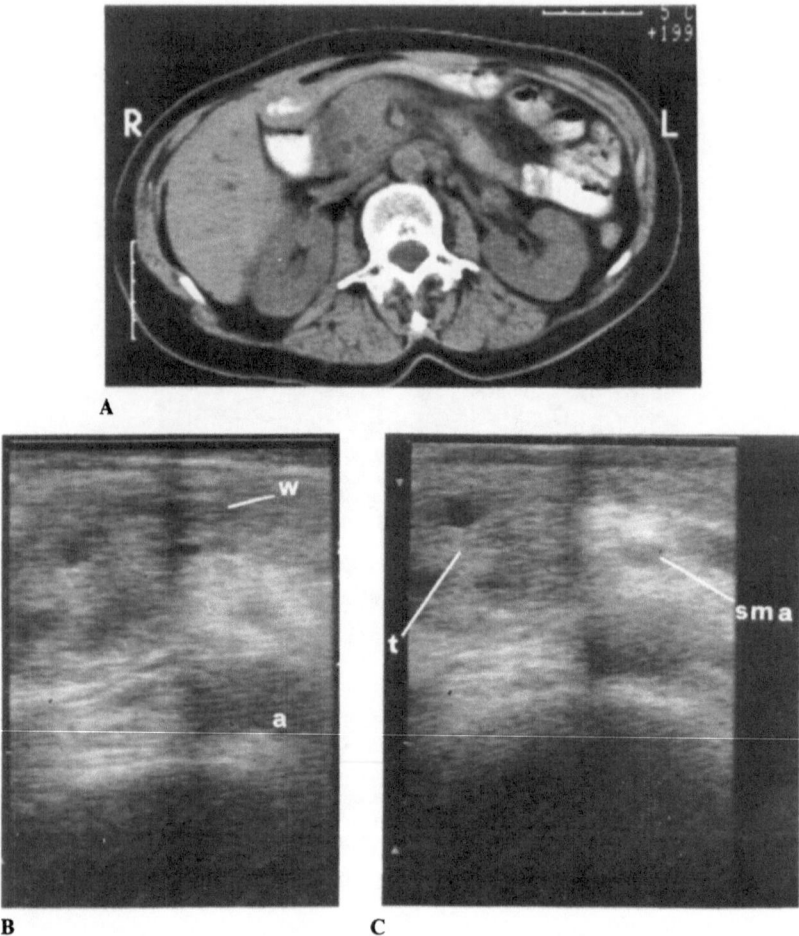

A

B   C

Figure 7.6. Pancreatic cystocarcinoma.
A) CT Scan shows a swelling in the head of the pancreas containing low-density lacunae.
B, C) Intraoperative ultrasound confirms this finding, showing an irregularly marginated mass with echo-spared lacunae filled with fluid in the head of the pancreas. Proximally, a slightly dilated Wirsung duct (w) is visible. Pancreatectomy was not performed on account of lymph node metastasis.

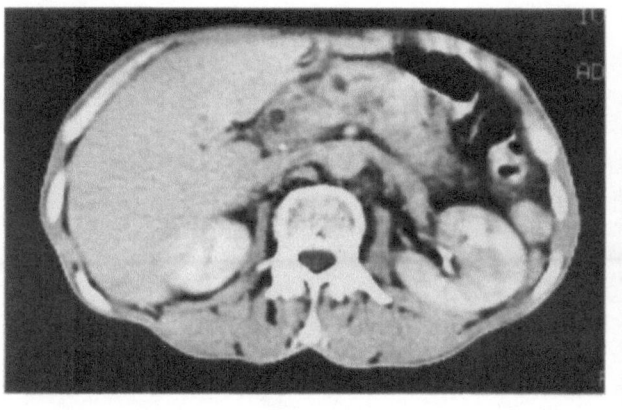

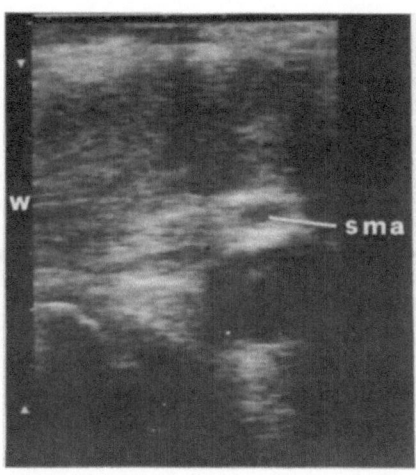

A

B

Figure 7.7. Chronic pancreatitis.
A) CT Scan shows an enlarged pancreas with low-density lacunae indicative of small cysts.
B) Intraoperative ultrasound shows a considerably enlarged pancreas with uneven echo-pattern. The Wirsung duct (w) near the head is normal size.

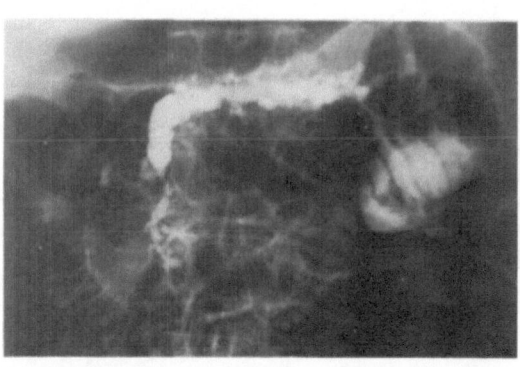

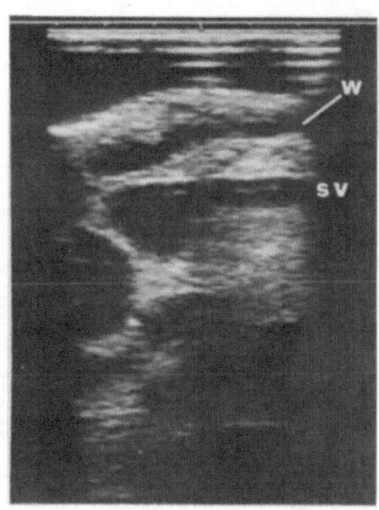

A   **B**

Figure 7.8. Chronic pancreatitis.
A) Retrograde Wirsung shows irregular dilatation of the Wirsung duct proximal to the cephalic stenosis.
B) Intraoperative echography, using a gel pad, shows the dilated Wirsung and also marked parenchymal atrophy.

144

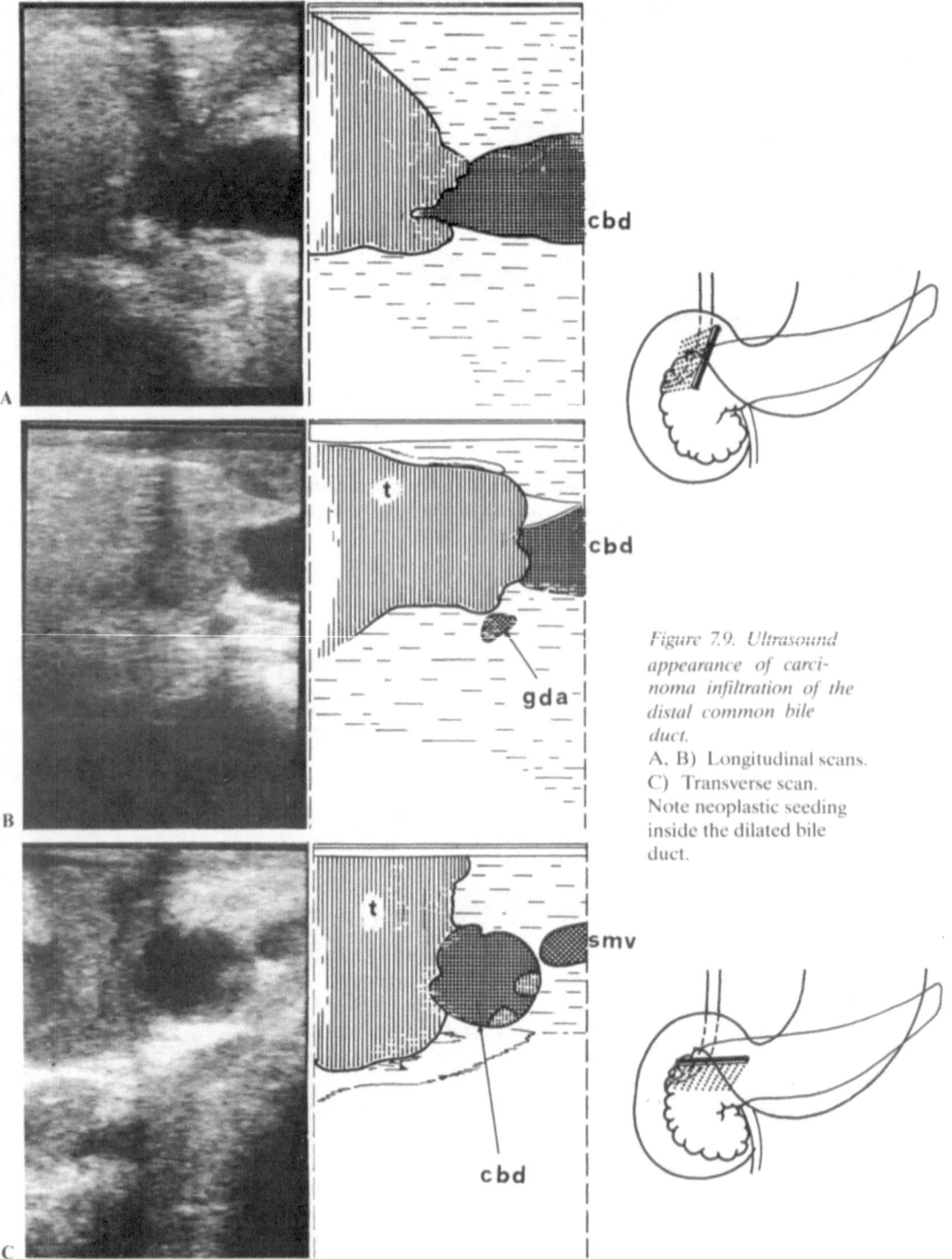

Figure 7.9. *Ultrasound appearance of carcinoma infiltration of the distal common bile duct.*
A, B) Longitudinal scans.
C) Transverse scan.
Note neoplastic seeding inside the dilated bile duct.

within the vessel (Fig. 7.9). Intraoperative ultrasound is often decisive in obstruction of the terminal portion of the common bile duct especially if preoperative investigations have failed to identify the nature of the obstruction. This, in fact, might be an embedded stone or cancer of the pancreatic head adjacent to the papilla or an ampullary carcinoma. In the event of papillary neoplasm, the lesion will appear as a hyperechoic projection into the duodenal lumen (Fig. 7.10).

Having located the lesion, the operator must then turn to investigation of the contiguous anatomical structure and especially the superior mesenteric and portal vein. Their involvement or not will be vital in determining whether the case is operable without having to venture into the highly delicate task of dissecting peripancreatic tissue. In the healthy patient the mesenteric and portal veins are seen to expand and contract with breathing [7]. This characteristic may be lost if the tumor has invaded the vessel or there might be a visible breach in the echogenic wall indicating tumor spill-over into the lumen. Interpretation is more difficult if the tumor only lies against the vessel wall without actually infiltrating it (Fig. 7.11). Here scans at various inclinations should be performed in order to weed out any false images that may be produced by a particular beam projection [21, 40].

Finally intraoperative ultrasound provides substantive support in determining the presence of liver metastasis which may escape preoperative exploration, being at times indistinguishable on account of concomitant dilatation of the intrahepatic bile ducts (Figs. 7.12, 7.13).

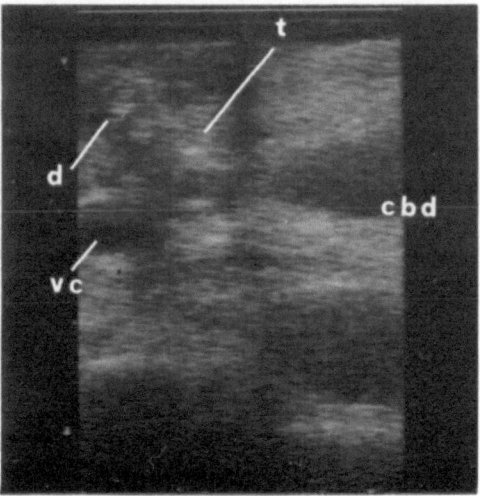

Figure 7.10. Neoplasia of the papilla. The common bile duct inside the pancreatic head is dilated. The tumor is the irregularly marginated, hyperechoic formation in the lumen of the duodenum.

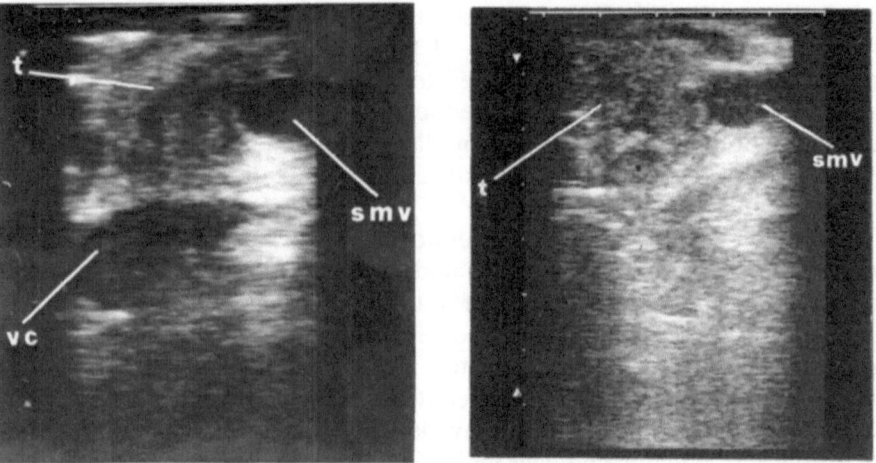

Figure 7.11. Neoplasms of the uncinate process of the pancreas. In both cases the tumor (t) appears closely connected to the superior mesenteric vein (smv). This ultrasonic picture always denotes vein wall infiltration despite the fact that the vein lumen is normal.

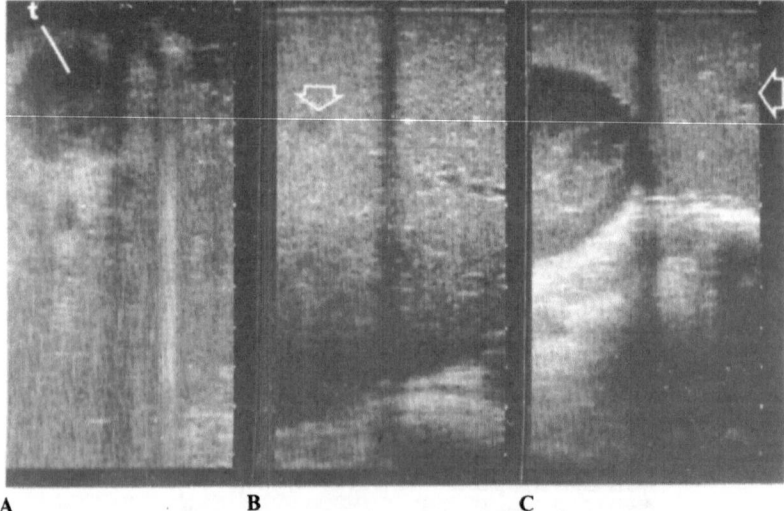

A   **B**   **C**

Figure 7.12. Tumor in the head of the pancreas (A) with small hypoechoic liver metastases (arrow) (B, C) missed at pre-operative ultrasound. There is sludge in the gallbladder due to bile obstruction.

Endocrine tumors

Among the endocrine tumors of the pancreas, insulinomas and gastrinomas are by far the most frequent and still today pose considerable diagnostic and management problems. On the diagnostic side, although hormone titers and

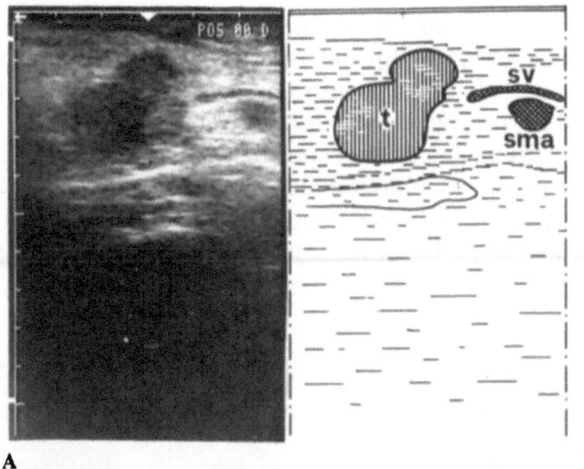

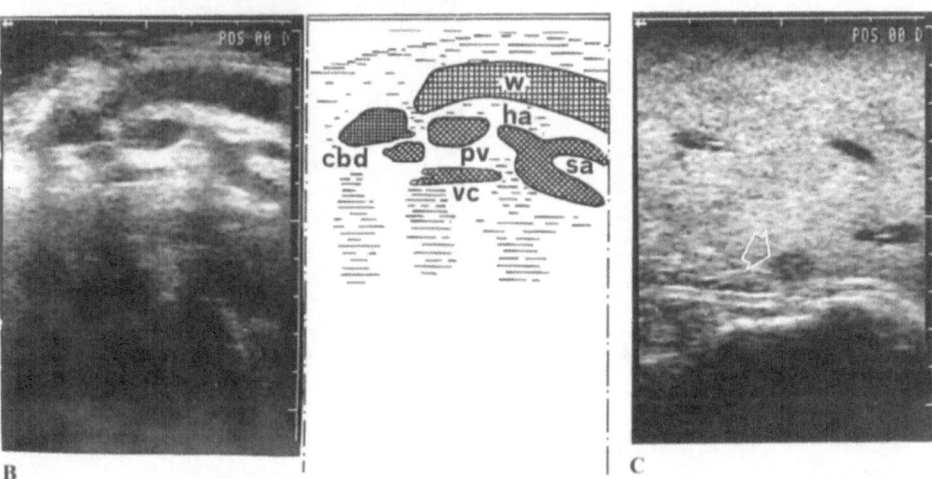

Figure 7.13. Pancreatic carcinoma with occult hepatic metastasis.
A, B) Tumor (t) measures 3 cm on its largest axis. Note proximity to the portal vein (pv) and
the superior mesenteric vein (smv) which respond to pressure exerted with the probe. The
tumor has caused dilatation of the Wirsung duct (w) and slight dilatation of the common bile
duct (cbd).
C) Inhomogeneous hypoechoic metastasis (arrow) of 9 mm in segment 8 of the liver.

stimulation tests do prove the presence of tumor, the exact location of the
lesion is not found either preoperatively or at surgery in some 1/3 of cases. In
fact insulinomas and gastrinomas are small – 0.3 to 2 cm – at times multifocal
(10% of insulinomas and 40% gastrinomas) or ectopic. Macroscopically they
are difficult to distinguish from pancreatic tissue, and 20 to 38% of all cases
are not palpated at surgery [1, 43, 44]. A similar percentage of tumors escapes
detection by preoperative work-up, due to the small size of the tumor and the

retroperitoneal position of the pancreas itself. Abdominal ultrasound scan picks up less than 30% of all insulinomas [17], at times missing tumors of 3 cm, and less than 20% of all gastrinomas [6]. CT scan does no better since both tumor and normal pancreatic tissue have the same density [12, 14]. Arteriography, although having greater specificity especially in detecting insulinomas, which are more vascularized [20, 27, 29], nonetheless gives numerous false negative results in the case of small tumors. Furthermore arteriography is of doubtful use in gastrinomas since these are often poorly vascularized

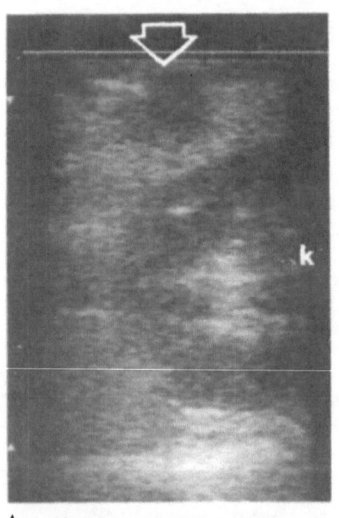

A

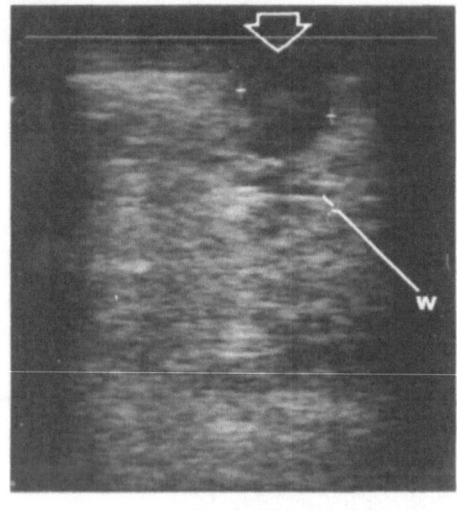

B

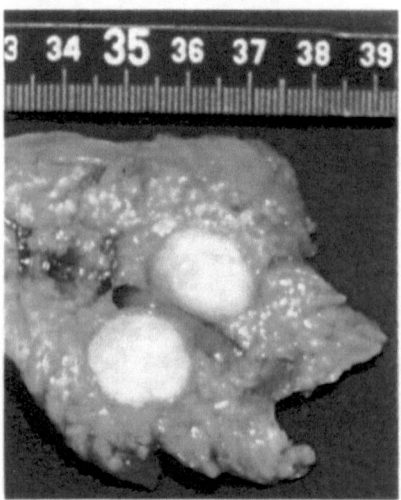

C

Figure 7.14. Insulinoma of the tail of the pancreas.

A) The tumor (arrow) appears as a small (12 mm) hypoechoic formation projecting anteriorly towards the left kidney. The lesion had not been picked up by radiological studies (CT Scan, angiography) nor at preoperative ultrasound.

B) At greater magnification, tilting the probe cranially, the lesion can be seen together with the Wirsung duct (w).

C) Operative specimen: distal pancreatectomy of the tail.

[23]. Catherization of the splenic vein for serial hormone titration remains the most reliable method of diagnosing the smallest tumors (26, 29). Hormonal assays, although not simple to carry out, do however single out the malfunctioning organ, without of course indicating the exact location of the tumor (13, 20).

However, despite extensive use of a variety of preoperative diagnostic techniques, the actual site of more than 30% of all insulinomas and gastrinomas diagnosed remains undetected preoperatively while 20–25% of tumors cannot be palpated at surgery.

In these cases of unknown tumor site, surgery is a matter of guesswork. The usual approach is blind distal pancreatectomy with progressive pancreatic resection. This, however, is complicated by high morbidity and mortality [18, 28, 34, 43, 44] and very often does not result in successful ablation of the tumor [1].

In the light of the above, intraoperative ultrasound has become a key diagnostic technique in surgery for endocrine pancreatic tumors. Tumor appearance at intraoperative ultrasound is of a well defined, clearly marginated hypoechoic mass (Figs. 7.14, 7.15, 7.16). It may be near the surface of the gland which may, as a result present a distorted outline, or be embedded in the parenchyma of the pancreas to the point of compressing the splenic vein without, however, infiltrating it [2]. The intraoperative ultrasound appearance is very similar to the appearance of larger adenomas at transabdominal scan

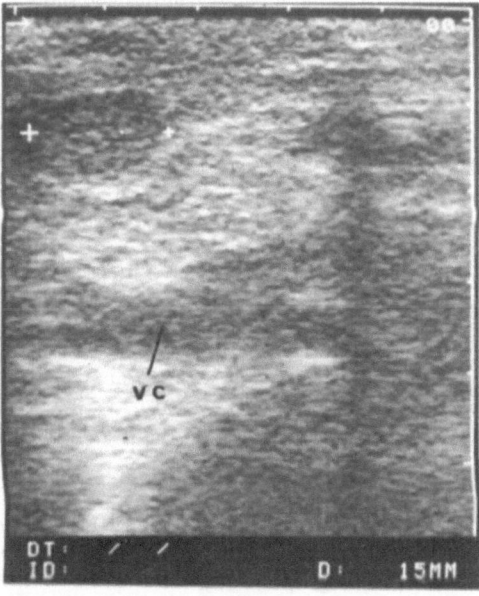

Figure 7.15. Small (15 mm) insulinoma of the head of the pancreas. Clinical examination and functional tests indicated a suspected lesion, which however was not detected preoperatively by ultrasound CT or angiography nor palpated at surgery.

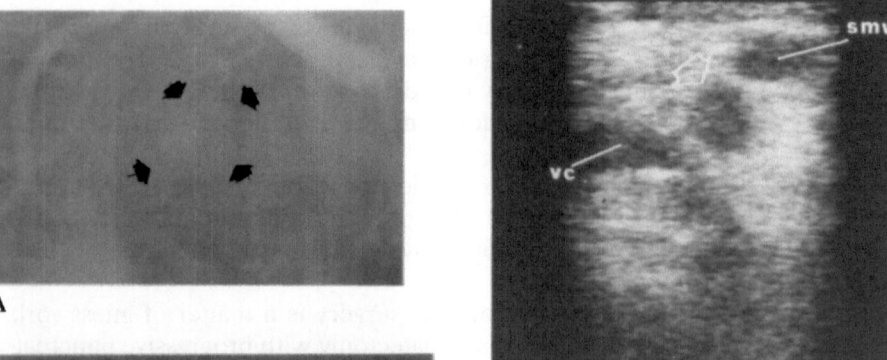

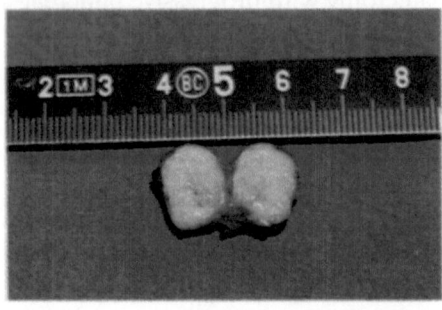

Figure 7.16. Insulinoma of the head of the pancreas. The lesion was identified at celiac arteriography as a hypervascularized mass in the head of the pancreas (A). At operation the lesion was not palpable inside the pancreatic head. Intraoperative ultrasound showed a hypoechoic nodule of 1.5 cm (arrow) in the uncinate proces of the pancreas between the superior mesenteric vein (smv) and the vena cava (B).
C) The tumor was enucleated after the head of the pancreas had been fully mobilized.

[9, 25, 37] or adenomas in other parts of the body [9]. Since its introduction, intraoperative ultrasound has indeed proved its worth, detecting tumors of even less than 1 cm [3, 4, 10, 11, 15, 16, 22, 23, 25, 33, 36, 39] which had been completely missed at surgical exploration [10, 30, 31, 37]. The advantages of being able to perform ablative surgery without recourse to blind pancreatic dissection requires no further comment.

Conclusions

Intraoperative ultrasound should be considered as complementary to both preoperative techniques such as CT scan, angiography, catherization of the Wirsung duct and other intraoperative methods such as direct visualization of the Wirsung duct and cholangiography. A judicious combination of these will provide the fundamental conditions for surgical success: accurate definition of the lesion, its nature and location vis-à-vis the surrounding vessels and ducts.

In the case of pancreatic carcinomas, intraoperative ultrasound supplies further information. Being able to immediately visualize the vascular structures allows appreciation of tumor resectability, while metastasis of the liver, not detected preoperatively, can be recognized easily even if the bile ducts are very dilated.

Finally, intraoperative ultrasound has proved especially useful in locating small endocrine tumors of the pancreas, rendering surgical procedure simpler, less random and more effective.

References

1. Adloff M., Ollier J. C., Cinqualbre J.: *Tumeurs langérhansiennes du pancréas.* Encyclopédie Médico-Chirurgicale, Paris. 7107, A 10, 2: 1–20, 1974.
2. Alexander J. H., Hernigou A., Billebaund M., Bouillot J. L., Merran S., Plainfossé M. C.: *Echotomographie per-opératoire en chirurgie pancréatique.* Lyon Chir. 80: 204–205, 1984.
3. Angelini L., Maceratini R., Bezzi M., Tucci G., Bonifacino A., Bezzi M., Ciulli A., Fegiz G.: *Intraoperative high resolution ultrasonography in the localization of occult pancreatic tumours.* Ital. J. Surg. Sci. 13,3: 209–215, 1983.
4. Angelini L., Bezzi M., Tucci G., et al.: *The ultrasonic detection of insulinomas during surgical exploration of the pancreas.* World J. Surg. 11: 642–647, 1987.
5. Boissel P., Porye C. H.: *Les tumeurs endocrines du pancréas.* Masson Ed., Paris, 1985.
6. Bollen E. C. M., Lawers C. B.: *Zollinger–Ellison syndrome due to a gastrin producing ovarian cystadenocarcinoma.* Br. J. Surg. 68: 776–8, 1981.
7. Bolondi L., Gandolfi L., Arienti V., Caletti G. C., Corcioni E., Gasbarrini G., Labò G.: *Ultrasonography in the diagnosis of portal hypertension: diminished response of portal vessel to respiration.* Radiology 142: 167–172, 1982.
8. Bolondi L., Gandolfi L., Labò G.: *Diagnostic ultrasound in Gastroenterology.* Piccin/Butterwords, Padova, 1982.
9. Chapuis Y., Hermigon A., Plainfosse M. C., Bonnette P.: *Exemples d'application de l'ultrasonographie temps réel peropératoire en chirurgie endocrinienne.* Chirurgie 110: 97–104, 1984.
10. Charboneau J. W., James E. M., Van Heerden J. A. et al.: *Intraoperative ultrasonographic localization of pancreatic insulinoma.* J. Ultrasound Med. 2: 251–4, 1983.
11. Cromack D. T., Norton J. A., Sigel B. et al.: *The use of high resolution intraoperative ultrasound to localize gastrinomas. An initial report of a prospective study.* World J. Surg. 11: 648–653, 1987.
12. Dumgaart-Petersen K., Stage J. G.: *CT scanning in patients with Zollinger-Ellison syndrome.* Scand. J. Gastroenterol. 43, 53: 117–122, 1979.
13. Doppman J. L., Brenman M. F., Dunnik N. R. et al.: *The role of pancreatic venous sampling on the localization of occult insulinoma.* Radiology 138: 557–62, 1981.
14. Dunnik N. R., Doppman J. L., Miller S. R., McCarthy D. M.: *Computed tomographic detection of pancreatic islet cell tumors.* Radiology 135: 117–120, 1980.
15. Gigot J. F., Gianello P., Dardenne A. N., Pringot J., Detry R., Otte J. B., Kestens P. J.: *Intraoperative ultrasonography in endocrine pancreatic surgery: preliminary results in 6 cases of insulinoma.* J.B.R.-B.T.R. 69: 57–62, 1986.
16. Gigot J. F., Detry R., Dardenne A. N., Pringot J., Otte J. B., Kestens P. J.: *Apport de l'échographie peropératoire en chirurgie pancréatique.* J.E.M.U. 8: 123–129, 1987.
17. Hancke S.: *Localization of hormone producing gastro-intestinal tumors by ultrasonic scanning.* Scand. J. Gastroenterol. 14, 56: 115–116, 1979.
18. Harrison T. S., Child C. G. et al.: *Current surgical management of functioning islet cell tumors of the pancreas.* Ann. Surg. 178: 485–495, 1973.

152

19. Ingemansson S., Kuhl C., Larsson L. J. et al.: *Localization of insulinomas and islet cell hyperplasia by pancreatic vein catherization and insulin assay.* Surg. Gynecol. Obstet. 146: 725–34, 1978.
20. Jensen R. T., Gardner J. T., Raufman J. P., Pandot S. J., Doppman J. L., Collen M. J.: *Zollinger-Ellison syndrome. Current concepts and management.* Ann. Int. Med. 98: 59–75, 1983.
21. Kasahara K., Yasuda Y., Fukomoto T. et al.: *Efficacy of intraoperative ultrasonography for vascular resection and reconstruction in surgery for pancreatic cancer.* Abstract n° 334; 1st World Congress Hepato-Pancreatico-Biliary, Surgery, Lund, June, 1986.
22. Klotter H. J., Ruekter K., Kummorle F., Rathmund M.: *The use of intraoperative sonography in endocrine tumors of the pancreas.* World J. Surg. 11: 635–641, 1987.
23. Luhn F. P., Gunther R., Rucker K. et al.: *Demonstration of pancreatic islet cell tumors.* J. Clin. Ultrasound 10: 173–5, 1982.
24. Lane R. J., Glazer G.: *Intraoperative B mode ultrasound scanning of the extraepatic biliary system and pancreas.* Lancet 2: 343–347, 1980.
25. Lane R. J., Compland G. A. E.: *Operative ultrasonic features of insulinomas.* Am. J. Surg. 144: 585–589, 1982.
26. Ludnerquist A., Erikson M., Ingemanson S., Larsson L. I., Reichardt W.: *Selective pancretic vein catheterization for hormone assay in endocrine tumors of the pancreas.* Cardiovasc. Radiol. 1: 117–124, 1978.
27. Marrano D.: *Ecografia Intraoperatoria, valori e limiti in chirurgia generale.* Arch. Societa Italiana Chirurgia, Masson It. Ed. 497–576, 1986.
28. Mengoli L., Le Duesme L. P.: *Blind pancreatic resection for suspected insulinoma: a review of the problem.* Br. J. Surg. 54: 749–56, 1967.
29. Moreaux J.: *Traitment chirurgical du syndrome de Zollinger-Ellison. Les résultats chez 34 malades.* Chirurgie 107: 557–565, 1981.
30. Norton J. A., Sigel B., Baker A. R. et al.: *Localization of an occult insulinoma by intraoperative ultrasonography.* Surgery 97: 381–3, 1985.
31. Norton J. A., Cromack D. T., Shawker T. H. and others: *Intraoperative ultrasonographic localization of islet cell tumors.* Ann. Surg. 207: 160–168, 1988.
32. Plainfosse M. C., Bouillot J. L., Rivaton F., Vaucamps P., Hernigou A., Alexandre J. H.: *The use of operative sonography in carcinoma of the pancreas.* World J. Surg. 11: 645–658, 1987.
33. Rifkin M., Weiss S. M.: *Intraoperative sonographic identification of nonpalpable pancreatic masses.* J. Ultrasound Med. 3: 409–413, 1984.
34. Schwartz S. S., Morwitz D. L., Zahfus B. et al.: *Continuous monitoring and control of plasma glucose during operation for removal of insulinomas.* Surgery 85: 702–4, 1979.
35. Shawker T. H., Doppman J. L., Dunnik N. R. et al.: *Ultrasonic investigations of pancreatic islet cell tumors.* J. Ultrasound Med. 1: 193–200, 1982.
36. Sigel B.: *Operative ultrasonography.* Lea and Febiger, Philadelphia, 1982.
37. Sigel B., Coelho J. C. U., Nyhus L. M. et al.: *Detection of pancreatic tumors by ultrasound during surgery.* Arch. Surg. 117: 1058–61, 1982.
38. Sigel B., Coelho J. C. U. et al.: *Ultrasonic assistance during surgery for pancreatic inflammatory disease.* Arch. Surg. 117: 712–716, 1982.
39. Siegel B., Duanie R., Coelho J. C. U., Nyhus L. M., Baker K. J., Machi J.: *Localization of insulinoma of the pancreas at operation by real time ultrasound scanning.* Surg. Gynec. Obstet. 156: 145–147, 1983.
40. Sigel B., Coelho J., Machi J., Flanigan D. P., Donahue P. E., Schulez J. J., Beitler J. C.: *The application of real time ultrasound imaging during surgical procedure.* Surg. Gynec. Obstet. 157: 33–37, 1983.
41. Sigel B., Machi J., Ramos J. R., Duarte B., Donahue P. L.: *The role of imaging ultrasond during pancreatic surgery.* Ann. Surg. 200: 486–493, 1984.

42. Sigel B., Machi J., Kikuchi T., Anderson K. W., Horrow M., Zaren H. A.: *The use of ultrasound during surgery for complications of pancreatitis.* World J. Surg. 11: 659–663, 1987.
43. Stefanini P., Carboni M., Patrassi N., Basoli A.: *The surgical treatment of occult insulinomas: a review of the problem.* Br. J. Surg. 61: 1–4, 1974.
44. Stefanini P., Carboni M., Patrassi N. et al.: *Beta cell tumors of the pancreas. Results of a study of 1067 cases.* Surgery 75: 597–601, 1974.

Chapter 8: Operative ultrasonography and endocrine tumors of the pancreas

Y. CHAPUIS*

Probably intraoperative ultrasonography is used to greatest profit in the detection of small endocrine tumors of the pancreas: insulinomas and gastrinomas. These are small, often multiple formations that preoperative investigations (ultrasound, CT scan, selective arteriography, selective venous catheterization), which are not without risk, fail detect.

In fact some 38% of all insulinomas are not detected prior to surgery. Of these 12 to 25% are either so small or deeply located as to escape detection at surgical exploration. Furthermore, even if a tumor is picked up, there is always the risk of missing a second, smaller nodule. Gastrinomas are even more difficult to identify since they are often multifocal and usually always small in size. The other endocrine tumors are too rare for any meaningful conclusions to be drawn as to the usefulness of intraoperative ultrasound as a diagnostic tool. Moreover these types of tumors are for the most part larger than 2 cm and hence easily palpable, thus obviating the need for intraoperative ultrasound.

The use of intraoperative ultrasound for the detection of endocrine tumors is more recent than in the case of exocrine tumors or chronic pancreatitis, with initially only anecdotal reports of findings [13, 28, 30].

Subsequently, however, reports of small lesions being detected by intraoperative ultrasound have appeared in the literature so that today accurate assessment is feasible of this method's usefulness and possible drawbacks.

Technique for the detection of endocrine tumors

The same real time ultrasound technique is adopted as for exocrine tumors or pancreatitis. Either a 7.5 or 10 MHz probe may be used, although the latter is somewhat less easy to handle. The probe can be wrapped in a sterile plastic bag and methyl cellulose gel used to ensure contact with the anatomical part. Otherwise the sterilized probe may be placed directly on the pancreas once the abdominal cavity has been filled with saline. When the pancreas appears normal without adhesions or distortions due to tumor, exploration is easy if the gland is exposed. From the tail to the isthmus of the pancreas, sagittal or longitudinal scans are most effective as they afford imaging of the aorta, the

* Clinique Chirurgicale de l'Hôpital COCHIN, 27 Rue du Faubourg Saint-Jacques, 75014 Paris.

splenic vein and further in depth, the point of entry of the inferior mesenteric vein and the superior mesenteric artery.

For the head of the pancreas, sagittal and transverse scans should be adopted, starting at the anterior face and proceeding laterally, placing the probe on the posterior face of the third portion of the duodenum facing the superior mesenteric branch. Any apparent anomaly should be examined from two planes since some appearances may resemble small lesions.

Investigation should be extended to the superior mesenteric and hepatic vessels and liver to detect possible metastases. Full mobilization of the head, using the Kocher maneouver, as well as the body and tail of the pancreas will enhance maneouvrability of the probe. However in order to avoid excessive detachment, dissection of the distal part of the gland should be avoided.

Results

There are several queries that must be answered concerning intraoperative sonography to detect endocrine tumors of the pancreas:
1. Is the ultrasound appearance of the adenoma(s) sufficiently characteristic or distinct as to be readily differentiated from surrounding healthy parenchyma, vessels or ductal structures?
2. Do the other lesions in or around the pancreas have a similar appearance?
3. What is the critical size or cut-off point for detection of lesions by the probe being used?
4. Has intraoperative ultrasonography picked up a lesion which escaped preoperative investigation as well as surgical exploration by a skilled professional?

   Although there is room for improvement and our experience must be furthered, the literature nonetheless does provide reports by 10 authors on this subject for a total of 55 insulinomas, 33 gastrinomas and 1 lipoma.
1. The ultrasound features of adenomas of the pancreas are similar to adenomas in other locations, i.e. a well marginated hypoechoic area that readily stands out from the surrounding pancreatic tissue which is more echogenic (Fig. 8.1, 8.2). This appearance is of course identical to that of adenomas detected at preoperative investigation. It affords differentiation from veins (hyperechoic walls, anechoic lumen, respiratory movements), arteries (hyperechoic walls, pulsatility), the Wirsung duct (thick, hyperechoic wall, anechoic lumen). A clearly visible delimitation of the hypoechoic zone would seem to suggest a benign lesion. However Norton [17] has recently shown that in the case of gastrinomas, poor demarcation of the hypoechoic area and ramifications into the pancreatic parenchyma is a sign of malignancy.
2. In the author's experience the only lesion presenting a similar appearance and which induced us erroneously to surgery, was an accessory spleen located in the pancreas (Fig. 8.3).

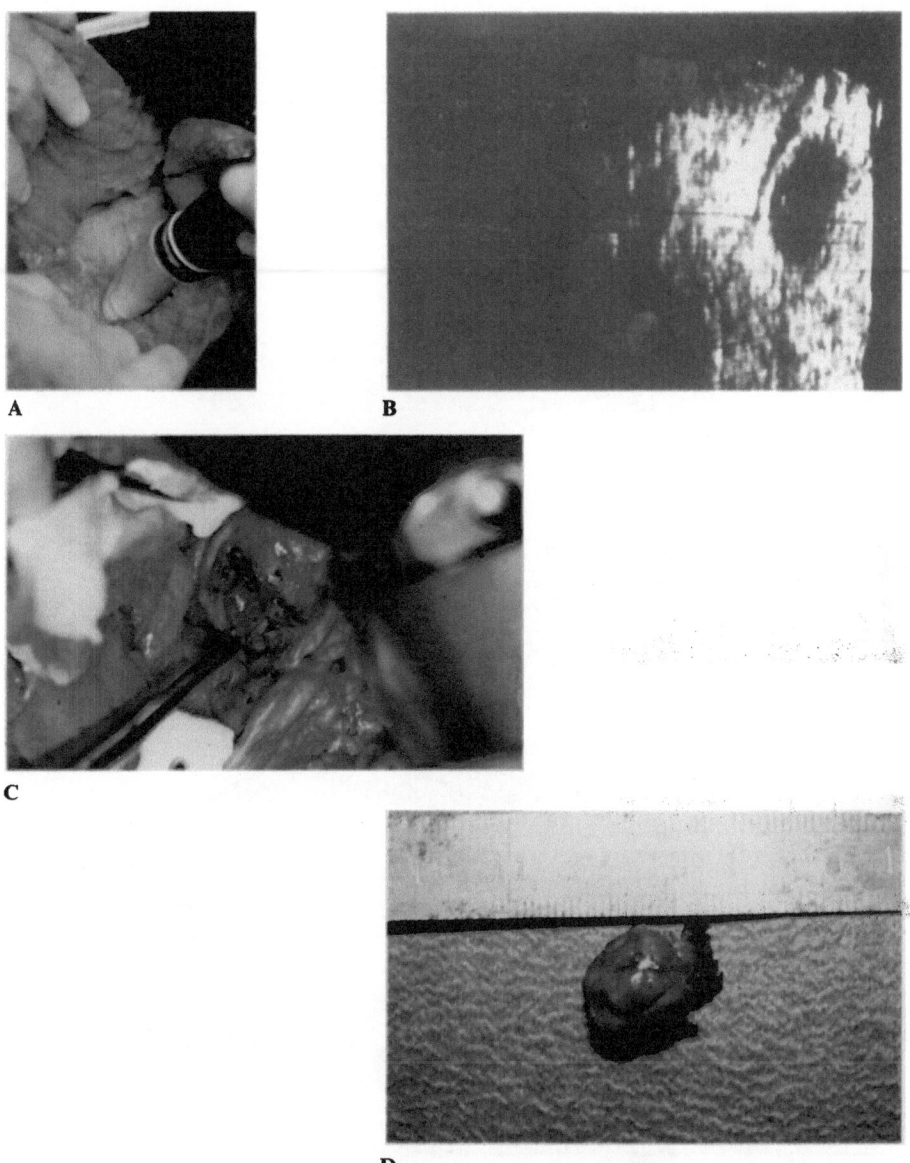

Figure 8.1. Search for an insulinoma located at the junction between the isthmus and head of the pancreas.

A) 7.5 MHz EDAP sectorial probe, a transverse scan.

B) Ultrasonic appearance of the insulinoma ($12 \times 12 \times 16$ mm).

C) Intraoperative view of the adenoma after incision of the pancreatic parenchyma.

D) The lesion after enucleation.

158

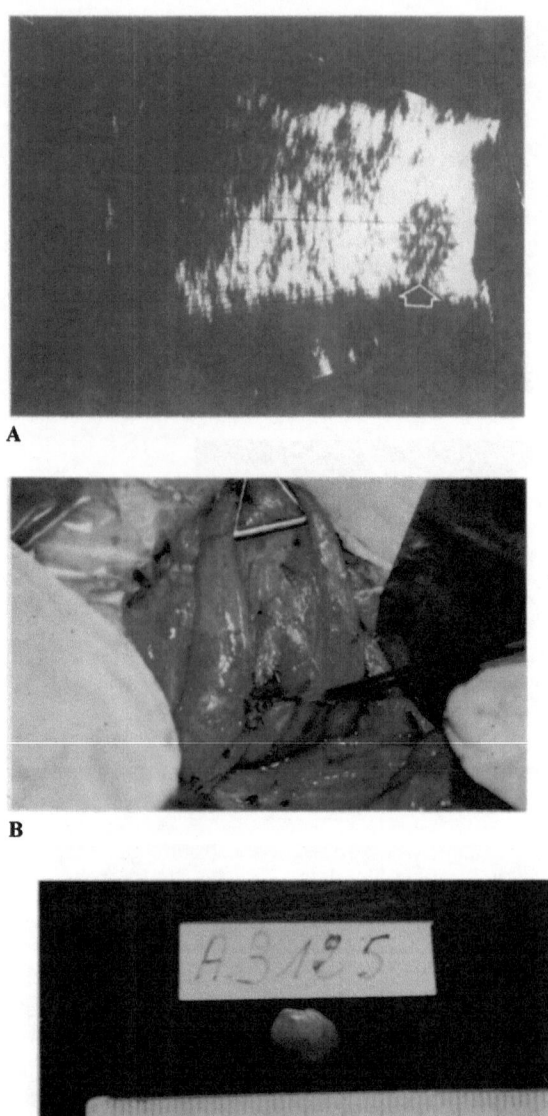

Figure 8.2. Pancreatic Gastrinoma.
A) Ultrasonic appearance: the hypoechoic lesion (arrow) impinges upon the duodenum on the posterior surface of the pancreas.
B) Operative field after duodeno-pancreatic detachment.
C) Operative specimen.

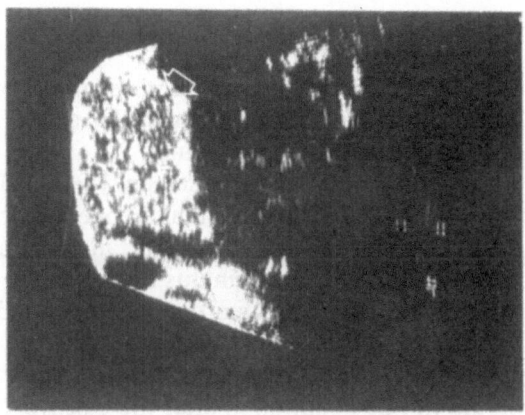

Figure 8.3. A false image of an adenoma in a patient with Zollinger-Ellison syndrome (accessory spleen). Note the hypoechoic area inside the tail of the pancreas (longitudinal scan).

3. Intraoperative ultrasound has detected tumors of 4 mm diameter [3, 4]. Below this size the investigation is not reliable [8] since certain images are of difficult interpretation. No adenoma of 5 mm or more detected during preoperative work-up or at surgical exploration has ever been missed by intraoperative sonography.
4. There are, however, several reports, one of which using selective splenic vein catheterization [3, 4, 6, 19] in which despite negative preoperative examinations, an adenoma was evidenced at intraoperative ultrasound investigation. However, the adenoma was also identified at exploration during surgery.

    While there are few false positives in the case of insulinomas [17], Norton reports 8 out of 23 false positives for gastrinomas of the pancreas [17].
5. The importance of intraoperative ultrasonography might seem questionable since most reports indicate that apart from whether the adenoma was detected preoperatively, it was always picked up by a trained surgeon at surgery. However intraoperative ultrasound has shown up tumors that were not detected even at careful palpation of the pancreas [6, 8, 19]. On operating a 35 year old woman for systemic hypoglycemia caused by an insulinoma, Norton [16] could not locate the lesion even after careful exploration despite the fact that venous catheterization had confined the area to the head of the pancreas. Arterioportography, ultrasound and CT scan showed no pathology. Using a 10 MHz probe, an 8 mm diameter hypoechoic lesion was detected at intraoperative ultrasound together with its relation to the common bile duct and the superior mesenteric asrtery and vein. This adenoma ($0.8 \times 0.8 \times 0.5$) was enucleated following a 2 cm incision in the parenchyma. Peix et al. [19] also report a similar case.

Indications

1. *Insulinomas* are the most frequent of all endocrine tumors of the pancreas. That surgical exploration may be usefully flanked by a tool such as intra-operative ultrasound is borne out by the following:

1.1 Almost 70% of all adenomas are less than 15 mm. Distribution is equally divided between head and body-tail areas. While tumors of at least 10 mm only rarely escape detection if the body and tail section is mobilized, lesions in the head or in the processus uncinatus are known to be more diffi-cult to locate especially since they are often deeply embedded in the paren-chyma.

1.2 In 10% of cases these insulinomas have two or more sites of growth. Thus exploration should not be abandoned after the discovery of one tumor. In this context intraoperative ultrasound presents as a valid means of enabling full investigation of the pancreas, having already allowed detection of multiple adenomas which had not been seen at surgical exploration [4, 6].

This intraoperative technique takes on even greater importance when the pre-operative work-up reveals little.

Boissel and Proye [2] report that of their 195 cases, almost 40% of the adenomas were not detected by preliminary examinations: arterioportogra-phy, ultrasound, CT scan or even portal vein catheterization. These data sup-port the other findings that almost 25% of all insulinomas are not detected at careful surgical palpation, even if this figure may well fall to 15% in the case of highly skilled surgeons of long experience. The above points to the advisibil-ity of having a tool to aid investigation during surgery.

For insulinomas, peripheral hormone assays and serial hormone assays during surgery using radioimmunological methods have been made available. These techniques, however, have not proved better than selective portal catheterization carried out preoperatively and furthermore, require about 45 minutes. Hence the interest that intraoperative ultrasound elicits especially in the light of data in the literature and research by Boissel and Proye. These lat-ter have studied 315 cases. Pre-operative investigations were positive 195 times and the adenoma was palpable 180 times. Therefore 12 adenomas were not detected and preoperative tests were negative 120 times. At surgery 83 insulinomas were palpable, meaning that complementary techniques and surgical exploration had failed 18 times. Of these 18 cases, on 6 occasions blind dissection led to discovery of the insulinoma, while in the other 12 cases it did not. These figures give an eloquent picture of the usefulness of ultra-sonography. In their series of 6 cases, Norton et al. [17] report intraoperative ultrasound as having a sensitivity of 86% as against 71% for palpation. Intra-operative ultrasound has two further advantages – it allows for echo-guided biopsy if necessary and indicates the relationship of the adenoma to the pan-creatic vessels and Wirsung canal. Finally intraoperative ultrasonography does away with the need for extensive pancreatectomies especially in the case of undiagnosed transient hypoglycemia caused by lipid-lowering sulfamides [19].

2. In the case of *gastrinomas* intraoperative ultrasound is of much more evident use. Pre-operative investigations often divulge little. Celio-mesenteric arteriography in positive in only 10% of cases, tomodensitometry in 20 to 30% and routine ultrasound in only a disappointing 20%. Although portal and splenic catheterization does give better results of around 50%, it is, however, an invasive technique entailing a certain risk. Furthermore the radiography images do not always match the surgical findings. Again this situation points to the usefulness for surgeons of an accurate investigation tool. Unfortunately gastrinomas are very small tumors, often around 5 mm, most frequently multifocal (Fig. 8.4) only rarely single (20 to 30%) with distribution throughout the pancreas. The metastatic adenopathies that in 60% of cases

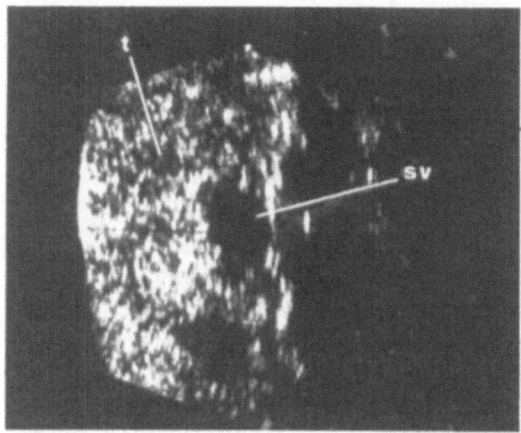

A

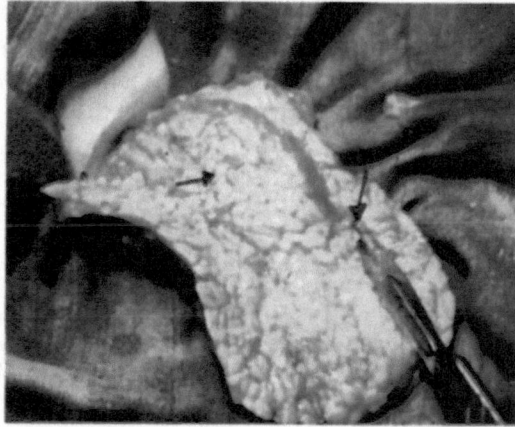

B

Figure 8.4. Small pancreatic gastrinomas detected at intraoperative ultrasound.
A) Small hypoechoic area (t) in the body of the pancreas. The gland presents a heterogeneous structure.
B) Appearance of a macroscopic adenoma which measured 5 mm on resection (caudal pancreatectomy). The second arrow indicates a further gastrinoma (4 mm).

accompany these lesion are fairly easy to palpate following extensive detachment of the pancreas. However, despite ease of identification in the majority of cases, diagnosis of duodenal or gastric gastrinomas would be greatly aided by the use of ultrasound. Of the 3 cases studied by us, only on one occasion did intraoperative ultrasound locate 2 adenomas of 4 and 6 mm in the body of the pancreas. In one case, the abnormal appearance turned out to be a supernumerary spleen and in the other case, while the pancreas was normal, the patient presented a completely invasive retro-duodenal adenopathy, which was also identified at intraoperative ultrasound. Pasquali [18], Ruckert [22], Sigel [28] and especially Norton [17] have published encouraging results. In our series of 2 gastrinomas of the pancreas, sensitivity was 95% for intraoperative ultrasound compared to 91% for palpation. If the lesion was outside the pancreas, however, sensitivity was only 58% as against 100% for palpation. In the light of the above, intraoperative ultrasound can be recommended during surgery for all types of Zollinger-Ellison syndrome.

Conclusion

While not infallible, intraoperative ultrasonography would today seem of considerable use during surgery for insulinomas, gastrinomas and apudomas in general. Initial results have been encouraging. It has the advantage of limiting pancreatic dissection in what often turns out to be futile exploration and enables continued search for other foci following ablation of the first adenoma. It also allows location of the vascular and other structures impinging upon the adenoma and thereby is a useful guide for the surgeon during resection.

Finally, if its promise if fulfilled, certain invasive techniques (percutaneous venous catheterization) or inconclusive investigations (pre-operative ultrasound and CT scans) may be avoided.

References

1. Angelini L., Maceratini R., Bezzi M., Tucci G., Bonifacino A., Bezzi M., Ciulli A., Fegiz G.: *Intraoperative high resolution ultrasonography in the localization of occult endocrine pancreatic tumors.* The Italian Journal of Surgical Sciences 13: 209–15, 1983.
2. Boissel P., Proye C.: *Les tumeurs endocrines du pancréas.* Masson, Paris, 1985.
3. Chapuis Y., Hernigou A., Poirier A., Luton J. P., Benali H.: *Detection of a pancreatic insulinoma by perioperative real time ultrasonography.* Presse Médicale 12: 40, 2535–2536, 1983.
4. Chapuis Y., Hernigou A., Plainfosse M. C., Bonnette P.: *Ultrasound imaging in real time during operation for endocrine surgery.* Chirurgie 110: 97–104, 1984.
5. Charbonneau J. W., James E. M., Van Heerden J. A., Grant C. S., Sheedy P. F.: *Intraoperative real-time ultrasonographic localization of pancreatic insulinoma: initial experience.* J. Ultrasound Med. 2 (6): 251–254, 1983.

6. Gigot J. F., Gianello P., Dardenne A. N., Otte J. B., Kestens P. J.: *L'échographie per-opératoire dans la chirurgie du pancréas endocrine: résultats préliminaires à propos de 6 insulinomes.* Gastro-entérol. Clin. Biol. 10: 219A, 1986.

7. Gunther R. W., Klose K. J., Ruckert K., Kuhn F. P., Beyer J., Klotter H. J., Cordes: *Islet cell tumors: detection of small lesions with computed tomography and ultrasound.*

8. Gunther R. W., Klose K. J., Ruckert K., Beyer J., Kuhn F. P., Klotter H. J.: *Localization of small islet cell tumors. Preoperative and intra operative ultrasound, computed tomography, arteriography, distal subtraction, angiography, and pancreatic venous sampling.* Gastrointest. Radiol. 10: 145–152, 1985.

9. Klotter H. J., Kuhn F. P., Ruckert K., Neher M., Hinkel E., Kummerle F.: *Intraoperative Ultraschalluntersuch bei Pancreaseingriffen.* Dtsch. Med. Wochenschr. 108: 1463–1468, 1983.

10. Kuhn F. P., Gunther R., Ruckert K., et al.: *Demonstration of pancreatic islet cell tumors.* J. Clin. Ultrasound 10: 173–175, 1982.

11. Lane R. J., Glazer G.: *Intraoperative B-mode ultrasound scanning of the extra hepatic biliary system and pancreas.* Lancet 2: 334–337, 1980.

12. Lane R. J.: *Intraoperative B-mode scanning.* J. Clin. Ultrasound 8: 334–337, 1980.

13. Lane R. J., Coupland G. A. E.: *Operative ultrasonic features of insulinomas.* Am. J. Surg. 144: 585–587, 1982.

14. Meran S., Plainfosse M. C., Alexandre J. H.: *L'échographie per-opératoire du pancréas.* Médicine et Chirurgie Digestive, 10: 6, 478, 1981.

15. Mouroux D., Aimino R., Brandone H., Nicolino J.: *Détection échographique pré-opératoire d'un insulinome.* Presse Méd. 13: 1963, 1984.

16. Norton J. A., Sigel B., Baker A. R., Ettinghausen S. E., Shawker T. H., Krudy A. G., Doppman J. L., Taylor S. L., Gordon P.: *Localization of an occult insulinoma by intraoperative ultrasonography.* Surgery 97: 381–384, 1985.

17. Norton J. A., Cromack D. T., Shawker T. H., Doppman J. L., Comi R., Gordon P., Maton P. N., Gardner J. D., Jensen R. T.: *Intraoperative ultrasonography localization of islet cell tumors. A prospective comparison to palpation.* Ann. Surg. 207: 2, 160–168, 1988.

18. Pasquali C., Rubaltelli L., Sperti C., Petrin C., Alfano A., Pedrazzoli S.: *Peroperative sonography in pancreatic apudomas. 31me Congrès de la Société Internationale de Chirurgie, Paris, 1985.* Abstruct, p. 639.

19. Peix J. L., Bel J. C., Maillet P. J., Lasras V., Fleury M. C.: *Chirurgie écho-guidée de l'adénome langheransien.* Lyon Chir. 83: 5, 357–359, 1987.

20. Plainfosse M. C., Merran S.: *Work in progress: intraoperative abdominal ultrasound.* Radiology 147 (3): 829–832, 1983.

21. Rifkim M. D., Weiss S. M.: *Intraoperative sonographic identification of non palpable pancreatic masses.* J. Ultrasound Med. 3: 409–411, 1984.

22. Ruchert K., Gunther R., Klotter H. J., Kummerle F.: *Intraoperative sonographische Localisation von Insulinomes.* Chirurg. 54: 589–591, 1983.

23. Rueckert K. F., Klotter H. J., Kummerle F.: *Intraoperative ultrasonic localization of endocrine tumors of the pancreas.* Surgery 96: 1045–1047, 1984.

24. Shawker T. H., Doppman J. L., Dunnickn R. et al.: *Ultrasonic investigation of pancreatic islet cell tumors.* J. Ultrasound Med. 1: 193–200, 1982.

25. Sigel B.: *Ultrasonography during pancreatic surgery. In: Operative Ultrasonography.* Lea & Febiger, Philadelphia, 85–109, 1982.

26. Sigel B., Coelho J. C., Donahue P. E., Nyhus L. M., Spigos D. G., Baker R. J., Machi J.: *Ultrasonic assistance during surgery to pancreatic inflammatory disease.* Arch. Surg. 117: 712–716, 1982.

27. Sigel B., Coelho J. C., Nyhus L. M., Velasco J. M., Donahue P. E., Wood D. K., Spigos D. G.: *Detection of pancreatic tumors by ultrasound during surgery.* Arch. Surg. 117: 1058–1061, 1982.

28. Sigel B., Duarte B., Coelho J. C., Nyhus L. M., Baker R. J., Machi J.: *Localization of insuli-nomes of the pancreas at operation by real-time ultrasound scanning.* Surg. Gynecol. Obstet. 156: 145–14729, 1983.
29. Sigel B., Coelho J. C., Machi J., Flanigan D. P., Donahue P. E., Schuler J. J., Bettler J. C.: *The application of real-time ultrasound imaging during surgical procedures.* Surg. Gyn. Obstet. 157: 33–37, 1983.
30. Sigel B., Machi J., Ramos J. R., Duarte B., Donahue P. E.: *The role of imaging ultrasound during pancreatic surgery.* Ann. Surg. 200: 486–493, 1984.
31. Sigel B., Machi J., Anderson K. W., Samuel S. P., Malik S. A., Haq S. Z., Duarte B., Dona-hue P. E., Baker R. J.: *Operative sonography of the biliary tree and pancreas.* Sem. Ultra-sound, CT and MR 6: 2–14, 1985.
32. Weill F.: *L'ultrasonographie en pathologie digestive.* Vigot Editeur, 1985.

Chapter 9: Intraoperative ultrasound during surgery for portal hypertension and liver transplantation

Intraoperative ultrasound investigation during shunt surgery for portal hypertension can provide the following:
- visualization of the vessels of the portal system and thus detection of thrombi or anatomical anomalies;
- location of vessels, especially the peripheral branches, which facilitates surgical manouvers;
- demonstration of the patency of the shunt;
- identification of any carcinomatous nodules in a cirrhotic liver.

Venous thrombosis

Although generally considered a rare event in cirrhotics [9], thrombi of the portal vein nonetheless present in about 10% of patients undergoing surgery for portal hypertension [1, 6, 10, 11]. Transabdominal ultrasound is more sensitive than arteriography in screening for portal thrombi, which are often parietal and do not completely obstruct the lumen [3]. The sensitivity of this preoperative technique is, however, severely impaired in the presence of meteorism or ascites.

Venous thrombosis presents with a variety of ultrasonic appearances depending on its size and age. Partially obstructive thrombi present as blocks of irregular echoes that give a distorted image to the wall and occupy part of the vessel lumen. In the case of an occlusive thrombus, the normal echo-spared tubular appearance of the vessels becomes hyperechoic, with on occasion poor delineation of the vessel walls. Recently formed thrombi are much less echogenic than long-standing thrombi.

Of 20 patients undergoing vascular surgery for portal hypertension, 2 were found to have venous thrombosis. One patient (Fig. 9.1) was being operated for recurrence of bleeding esophageal varices despite previous sclerosing therapy carried out endoscopically. Arteriography had not detected any portal anomaly. At intraoperative ultrasound, however, irregular echoes were seen in the portal branch, testifying to a non-occlusive thrombus. The resultant surgery was a distal spleno-renal anastomosis according to the Warren technique. The second was an emergency case of ruptured esophageal varices (Fig. 9.2). Intraoperative ultrasound showed a thrombus in the vena cava as well as a hepatocarcinoma of the 6th segment, both of which had not been picked up by preoperative ultrasound. In the event, surgery consisted of es-

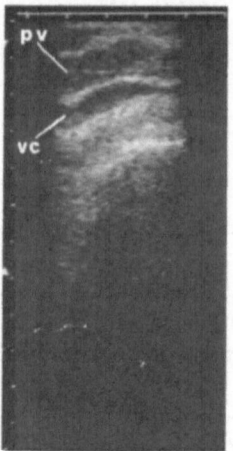

Figure 9.1. Thrombus in the portal vein. Irregular, low level echoes are visible in the vessel lumen. Typical image of a recently formed thrombus.

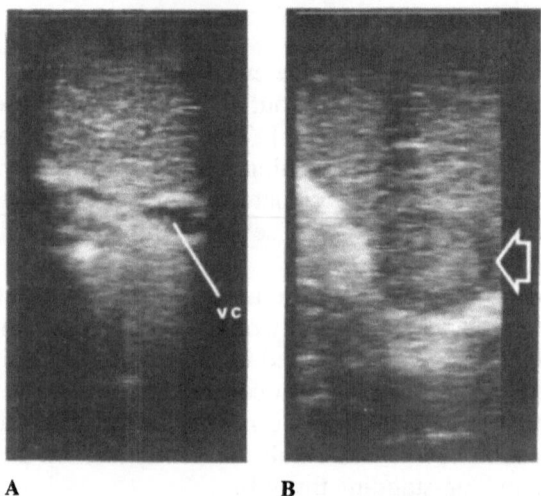

A　　　　　　　　B

Figure 9.2. Vena cava thrombosis (A) with concomitant hepatocarcinoma of the 6th segment (B).

ophageal transection rather than the portocaval anastomosis that had been planned.

Vascular mapping

Intraoperative ultrasound is especially useful to the surgeon in pin-pointing the actual location of the vessels that are candidates for anastomosis. The result is a more circumscribed surgical dissection, particularly in the case of peripheral shunts such as mesenteric-caval anastomosis [5, 13] and when performing a Warren-type procedure. Moreover, patients with portal hypertension also have severe liposclerosis of the mesos and retroperitoneum which is concomitant with hypertrophy of the lymphatics that in turn causes often abundant lymphatic effusion [2].

With intraoperative ultrasound, one can ascertain the exact vessel course (Fig. 9.3), distance from the surface, proximity of other structure and the distance between the vessels to be anastomized (Fig. 9.4). The resultant economy of dissection for exploration cuts theatre time considerably. Anatomical anomalies are clearly evidenced, such as a right hepatic artery deriving from the superior mesenteric artery.

Checking shunt patency

Patency of the anastomosis and correct positioning of the vessels (Figs 9.5 and 9.6) can be ascertained by intraoperative scan; correctly orienting the probe will image both the lumen of the anastomosis and the blood flowing through the vessels.

Search for hepatocarcinoma nodules

Hepatocarcinoma is an all too frequent sequela in the natural history of cirrhosis of the liver [7, 8], especially subsequent to hepatitic cirrhosis, which makes up the majority of our case material. 2 out of 20 patients undergoing surgery for portal hypertension were found to have a cancerous nodule that

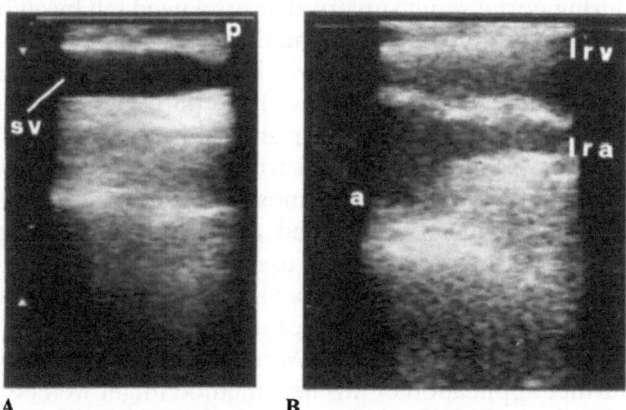

A   B

Figure 9.3.
A) *Normal splenic vein* observed with probe resting on the tail of the pancreas. The vein courses approximately 1 cm below the probe.
B) *Overview of the left renal vessels.*

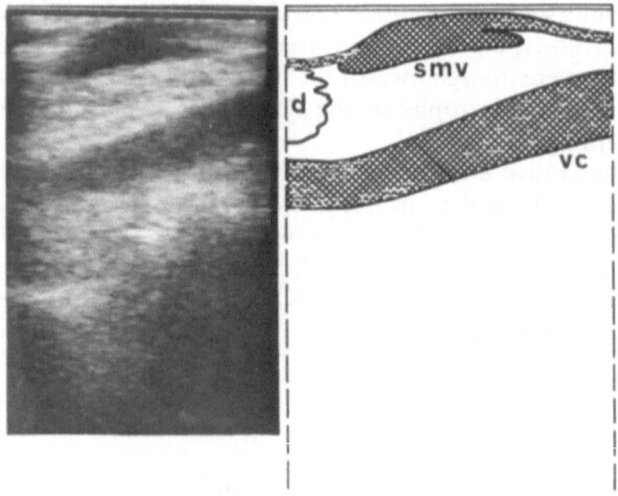

Figure 9.4. Layout of the superior mesenteric vein and the vena cava. The two vessels are about 2 cm apart.

had escaped detection at angiography and pre-op. scan and furthermore, was not palpable at surgery. In the first case (Fig. 9.7) the nodule (2.5 cm) was under the dome and in the second case (Fig. 9.2) it was in the posterior portion of the 6th segment and concomitant with thrombosis of the inferior vena cava.

As well as these morphological findings, it is now possible using Doppler ultrasound equipment to study blood flow. The pertinence of this method in the planning and control of shunt surgery is self-evident. Being able to assess blood flow during portal shunt surgery answers a need felt by all practicioners to carry out 'more physiologic' reconstruction respecting the particular hepato-portal circulation of the cirrhotic liver [10]. In fact several hemodynamic studies both pre and post operative, have been published. Depending on the study, either portal hepatic flow [12] or arterial hepatic flow [4] are seen as being of major importance. Flow measuring methods vary, however; direct measurement of flow is certainly the most reliable method but this means applying electromagnetic probes around the vessels, something that is not always feasible during surgery [10]. The use of Doppler ultrasound or Duplex systems during surgery affords flow readings of other vessels as well as the anastomosed area without having to resort to tissue dissection. Figure 9.8 gives the Doppler flow tracing for a Warren-type distal spleno-renal anastomosis. A further application of this new method might well be to check the various anastomoses – especially portal and arterial – performed during liver transplant surgery [14].

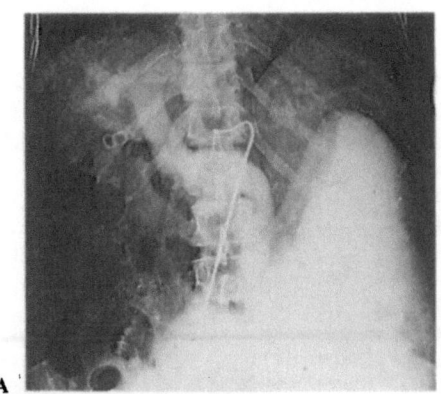

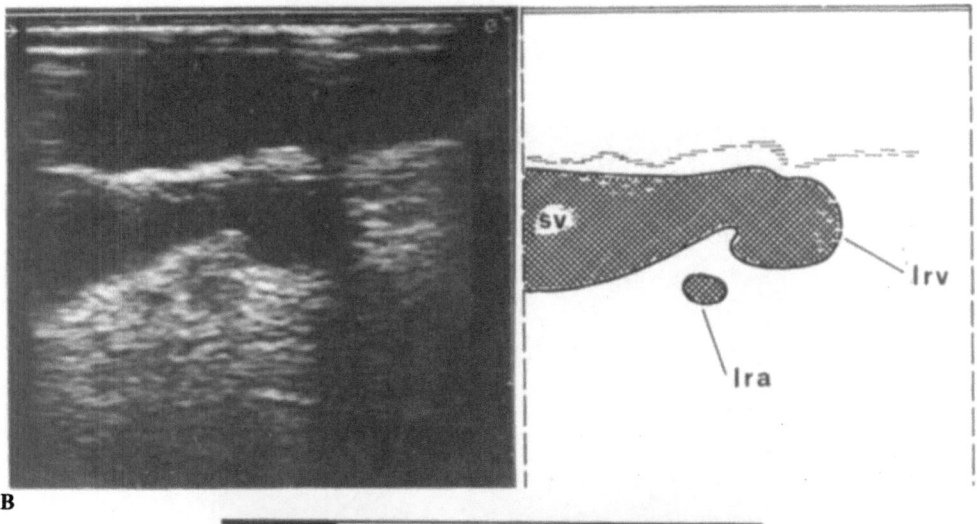

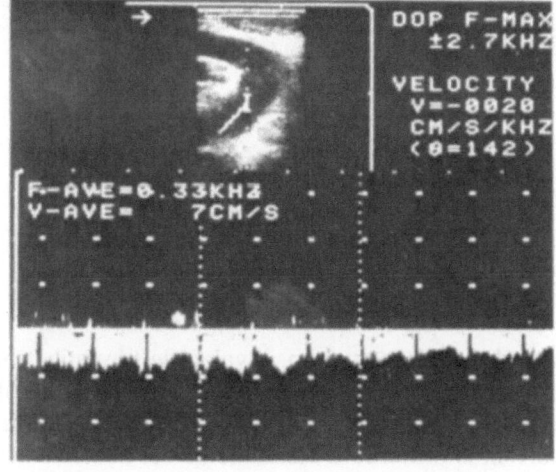

Figure 9.5. Conventional spleno-renal anastomosis. This procedure is now used in special cases only, such as this patient with an enormous splenomegaly (A) associated with hypersplenism and a history of bleeding esophageal varices. To demonstrate patency of the anastomosis with US, the probe must be 'flooded' with saline. (B). The Doppler ultrasound tracing shows good flow towards the left renal vein. (C).

170

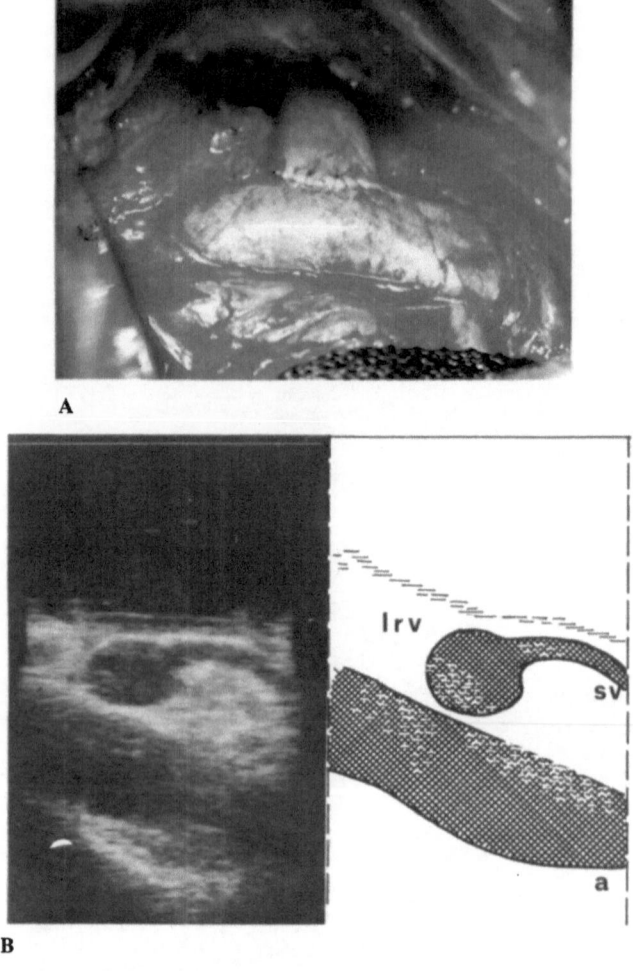

Figure 9.6.
A) *Distal spleno-renal anastomosis.*
B) *Longitudinal scan,* using the 'flooding' technique.

Intraoperative duplex ultrasound in liver transplantation

Duplex ultrasound has become an invaluable investigation technique in liver transplantation. In the preoperative work up patency of the recipient's portal vein and inferior vena cava can be assessed, showing hepatopetal flow when the portal vein is difficult to visualize or the absence of flow in cases of recent thrombosis and which go undetected by conventional real time imaging. Even more important is the role of Duplex ultrasound in the post-operative follow-up of patients undergoing liver transplant. Occlusion or

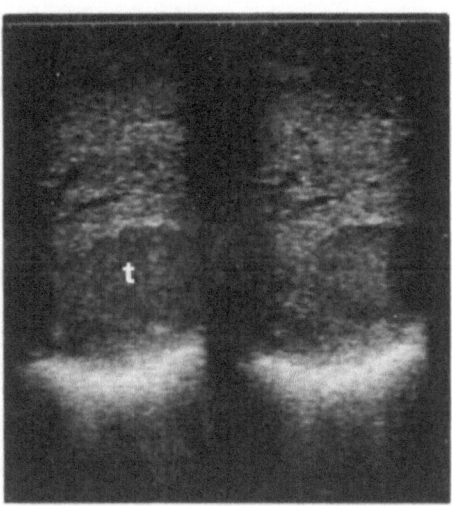

Figure 9.7. Occult hepatocarcinoma nodule in a cirrhotic liver, situated in the posterior portion of the 7th segment. The mass is hypoechoic without an outer halo.

stenosis of the hepatic artery is the most frequent vascular complication and its clinical presentation is often dramatic and may require emergency retransplantation. This may be diagnosed by Duplex ultrasound [14] when no arterial signals are detected at the porta hepatis or in the intrahepatic branches. Portal vein thrombosis and stenosis may also be revealed by Duplex examination when no flow or localized acceleration of flow are visualized.

There are no published data on the role of the intraoperative application of Duplex ultrasound in liver transplantation.

On the basis of our experience we believe that it may be of crucial importance in many instances since it can:

1. reveal partial thrombosis of the portal vein (Fig. 9.9), which may not be evidenced at pre-operative ultrasonographic or angiographic diagnosis. In these cases Duplex ultrasound can establish not only the level and extension of the mural thrombosis but also its hemodynamic consequences, i.e. if portal flow to the liver is significantly dampened or not (Fig. 9.10);
2. assess the patency of the vascular anastomosis, both of the portal vein (Fig. 9.11) and the hepatic artery (Fig. 9.12). This is particularly important when a complex reconstruction of hepatic arterial inflow has to be performed on account of anatomical variations (for example when the donor's branch of the hepatic artery originates separately from the aorta). In these cases the finding of a normal arterial Doppler signal at the level of the extrahepatic artery and its intrahepatic branches (Fig. 9.13) confirms the hemodynamic efficiency of the surgical anastomosis.

We believe that further applications of intraoperative Duplex ultrasound and comparison with the post-operative follow up will provide in-

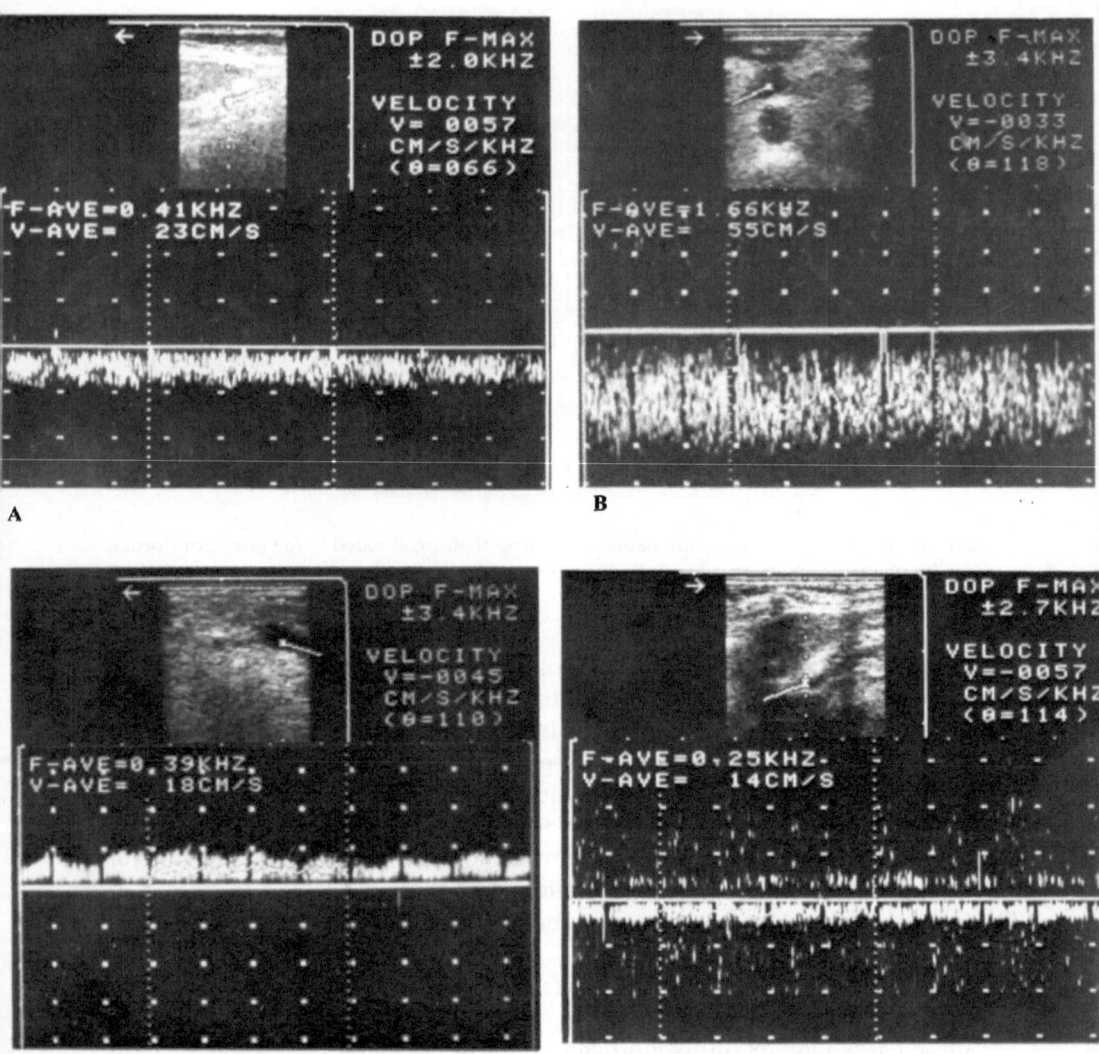

Figure 9.8. Doppler-flow studies during Warrenshunt.

A) Preoperative Doppler flow reading of the mesenteric portal circulation showing good flow to the liver (average velocity = 23 cm/s).

B) Rapid turbulent flow around the anastomosis.

C) The portal blood flow remains hepatopetal following surgery.

D) Doppler ultrasound of the portal mesenteric circulation 6 months post-operatively shows persistence of good portal hepatic perfusion (average velocity in the segment examined = 14 cm/s).

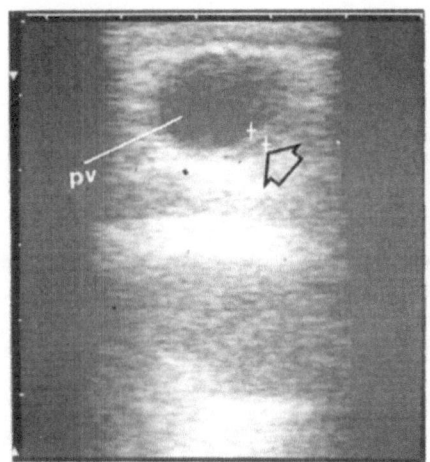 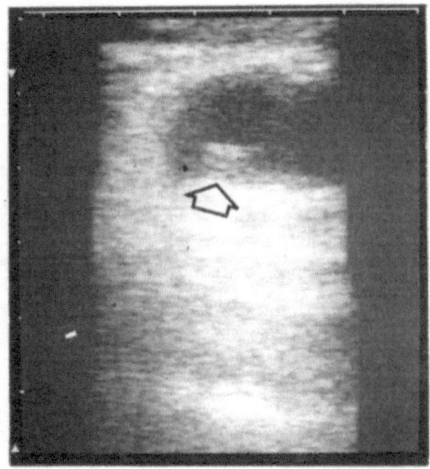

Figure 9.9. Intraoperative Duplex ultrasound during liver transplantation with a 5 MHz linear array transducer.
A) Transverse scan with a 5 MHz linear array transducer showing a thrombus (arrow) on the posterior wall of the portal vein (pv).
B) Oblique scan. The thickness of the thrombosis at this level is 3 mm and the lumen is not occluded.

teresting information of changes in hepatic hemodynamics following liver transplantation.

174

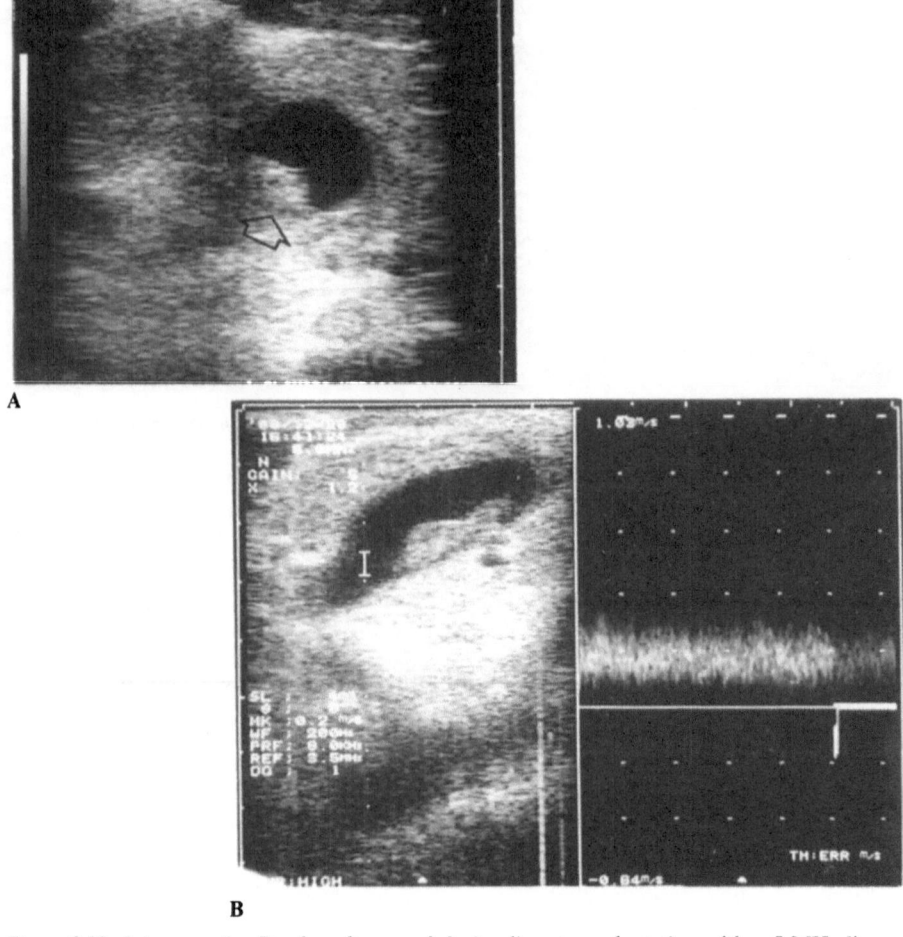

A

B

Figure 9.10. Intraoperative Duplex ultrasound during liver transplantation with a 5 MHz linear array transducer.
Transverse scan with a 5 MHz linear array transducer.
A) Transverse scan of the portal vein showing partial thrombosis (arrow) on the left posterior wall.
B) Longitudinal scan showing the extension of the thrombosis. Doppler analysis (on the right of the image) shows a normal hepatopetal flow.

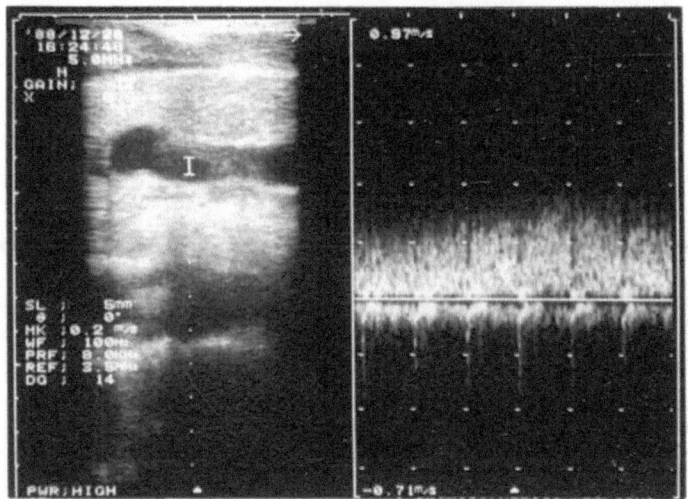

Figure 9.11. Intraoperative Duplex ultrasound of the portal vein during liver transplantation with a 5 MHz linear array transducer. The sample volume is positioned at the level of the surgical anastomosis and normal flow is displayed (right of the image).

References

1. Belli L., Sansalone C. V., Aseni P., Romani F., Rondinara G.: *Portal thrombosis in cirrhotics. A retrospective analysis.* Ann. Surg. 203: 286–291, 1986.
2. Bismuth H., Grange D.: *Dérivations portales sélectives.* Encycl. Méd. Chir., Paris. Techniques Chirurgicales. App. Dig. 40820: 4, 7, 12.
3. Bolondi L., Mazziotti A., Arienti V., Casanova P., Gasbarrini V., Cavallari A., Bellusci R., Gozzetti G., Possati L.: *Ultrasonographic study of portal venous system in portal hypertension and after surgical porto-systemic shunts.* Surgery 95: 261–269, 1984.
4. Burchell X. R., Moreno A. M., Panke W. F., Nealon T. F.: *Hemodynamic variables and prognosis following portocaval shunt.* Surg. Gynecol. Obstet. 138: 359–363, 1974.
5. Drapanas T.: *Interposition mesocaval shunt for treatment of portal hypertension.* Ann. Surg. 176: 435–447, 1972.
6. Fagner P., Saubier E., Brette R.: *Les obstructions portales.* Lyon Med. 687–798, 1974.
7. Liwa Y. F., Tai D., Chu C. et al.: *Early detection of hepatocellular carcinoma in patients with chronic type B hepatic.* Gastroenterology 90: 263–267, 1986.
8. Munoz N., Linsell A.: *Epidemiology of primary liver cancer.* In: *'Epidemiology of cancer of the digestive tract'* Ed. P. Correa, W. Haensel. Martinus Nijhoff Publ. (The Hague), 1982.
9. Okuda K., Ohnishi K., Kimura K. et al.: *Incidence of portal vein thrombosis in liver cirrhosis.* Gastroenterology 89: 279–286, 1985.
10. Possati L.: *Diagnostica dell'ipertensione portale.* Atti Soc. It. Chir. vol. I, 1974.
11. Sarjeh J.: *Portal vein thrombosis associated with cirrhosis: clinical importance.* Arch. Surg. 114: 902–905, 1979.
12. Steegmuller K. W., Marklin H. M., Hollis H. W.: *Intraoperative hemodynamic investigations during portacaval shunt.* Arch. Surg. 119: 269–273, 1984.
13. Stipa S., Ziparo V.: *Mesenterico-caval shunt.* In: *Medical and surgical problems of portal hypertension.* Ed. by Orloff, Stipa, Ziparo, Academic Press Inc. (London) 147–152, 1980.
14. Taylor K. G. W., Morse S. S., Weltin G. G., Riely C. A., Flye M. W.: *Liver transplant recipients: portable duplex US with correlative angiography.* Radiology 159: 357–363, 1986.

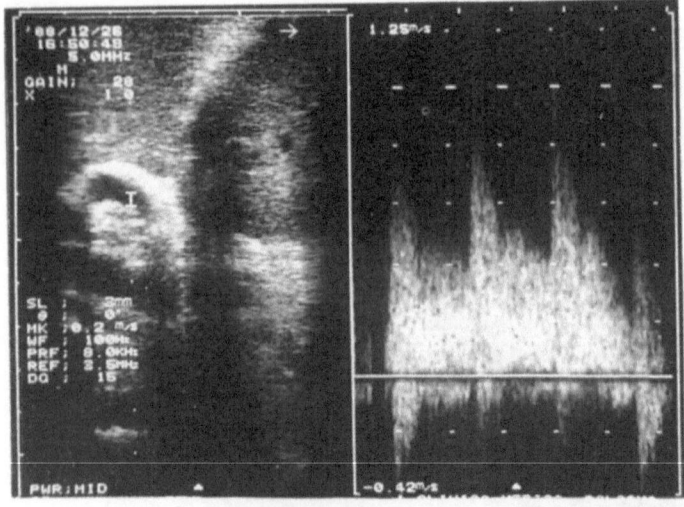

A

B

Figure 9.12. Intraoperative Duplex ultrasound of the hepatic artery during liver transplantation with a 5 MHz linear array transducer. The patency of the anastomosis is assessed by detecting the pulsating arterial signal at the level of the main trunk of the hepatic artery (A) and the right branch (B).

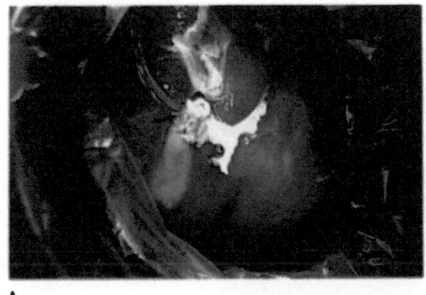

A

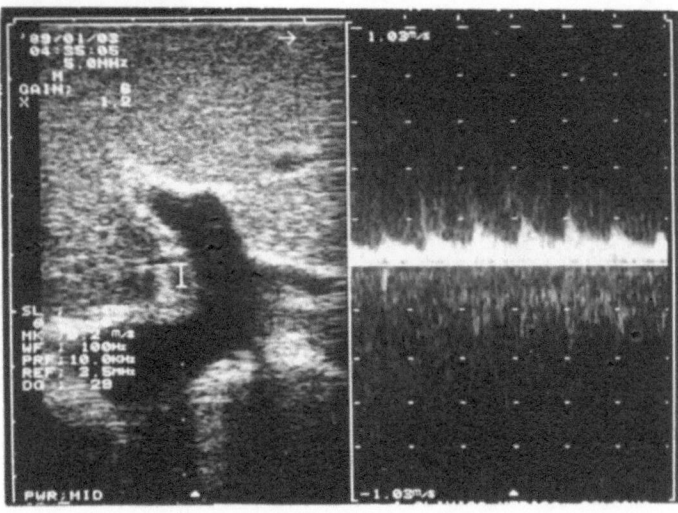

B

Figure 9.13. Intraoperative Duplex ultrasound of the hepatic artery during liver transplantation with a 5 MHz linear array transducer. In this case the left hepatic artery presented an independent origin from the aorta and a complex reconstruction of the arterial inflow to the liver was necessary (anastomosis of the left hepatic artery on the main hepatic trunk) (A). The success of the surgical reconstruction is demonstrated by the presence of an arterial signal on a branch of the left hepatic artery (B).

Index of Subjects

SERIES IN RADIOLOGY

1. J. O. Op den Orth: *The Standard Biphasic-contrast Examination of the Stomach and Duodenum*. Method, Results, and Radiological Atlas. 1979   ISBN 90–247–2159–8
2. J. L. Sellink and R. E. Miller: *Radiology of the Small Bowel*. Modern Enteroclysis Technique and Atlas. 1982   ISBN 90–247–2460–0
3. R. E. Miller and J. Skucas: *The Radiological Examination of the Colon*. Practical Diagnosis. 1983   ISBN 90–247–2666–2
4. S. Forgács: *Bones and Joints in Diabetes Mellitus*. 1982   ISBN 90–247–2395–7
5. Gy. Németh and H. Kuttig (eds.): *Isodose Atlas for Use in Radiotherapy*. 1981   ISBN 90–247–2476–7
6. J. Chermet: *Atlas of Phlebography of the Lower Limbs*. Including the Iliac Veins. 1982   ISBN 90–247–2525–9
7. B. K. Janevski: *Angiography of the Upper Extremity*. 1982   ISBN 90–247–2684–0
8. M. A. M. Feldberg: *Computed Tomography of the Retroperitoneum*. An Anatomical and Pathological Atlas with Emphasis on the Fascial Planes. 1983   ISBN 0–89838–573–3
9. L. E. H. Lampmann, S. A. Duursma and J. H. J. Ruys: *CT Densitometry in Osteoporosis*. The Impact on Management of the Patient. 1984   ISBN 0–89838–633–0
10. J. J. Broerse and T. J. Macvittie: *Response of Different Species to Total Body Irradiation*. 1984   ISBN 0–89838–678–0
11. C. L'Herminé: *Radiology of Liver Circulation*. 1985   ISBN 0–89838–715–9
12. G. Maatman: *High-resolution Computed Tomography of the Paranasal Sinuses, Pharynx and Related Regions*. Impact of CT Identification on Diagnosis and Patient Management. 1986   ISBN 0–89838–802–3
13. C. Plets, A. L. Baert, G. L. Nijs and G. Wilms: *Computer Tomographic Imaging and Anatomic Correlation of the Human Brain*. A Comparative Atlas of Thin CT-scan Sections and Correlated Neuro-anatomic Preparations. 1987   ISBN 0–89838–811–2
14. J. Valk: *MRI of the Brain, Head, Neck and Spine*. A Teaching Atlas of Clinical Applications. 1987   ISBN 0–89838–957–7
15. J. L. Sellink: *X-Ray Differential Diagnosis in Small Bowel Disease*. A Practical Approach. 1988   ISBN 0–89838–351–X
16. Th.H.M. Falke (ed.): *Essentials of Clinical MRI*. 1988   ISBN 0–89838–353–6
17. B. D. Fornage: *Endosonography*. 1989   ISBN 0–7923–0047–5
18. R. Chisin (ed.): *MRI/CT and Pathology in Head and Neck Tumors*. A Correlative Study. 1989   ISBN 0–7923–0227–3
19. G. Gozzetti, A. Mazziotti, L. Bolondi and L. Barbara (eds.): *Intraoperative Ultrasonography in Hepato-biliary and Pancreatic Surgery*. A Practical Guide. With Contributions by Y. Chapuis, J.-F. Gigot and P.-J. Kestens. 1989   ISBN 0–7923–0261–3
20. A. M. A. De Schepper and H. R. M. Degryse: *Magnetic Resonance Imaging of Bone and Soft Tissue Tumors and Their Mimics*. A Clinical Atlas. With Contributions by F. De Belder, L. van den Houwe, F. Ramon, P. Parizel and N. Buyssens. 1989   ISBN 0–7923–0343–1